Dr. S.

Medicinal Herbs & Treatments: *Heal Your Body from Diseases, strengthen your Immune System with Dr.Sebi's approved Herbs*

AMBER FLOREY

"If Nature didn't make it, don't take it"- **Dr. Sebi.**

Table of Contents

BOOK 1

BOOK 2

BOOK 3

Amber Florey

BOOK 1

INTRODUCTION

WHO IS DOCTOR SEBI?

"Healing has to be consistent with life itself. Suppose it isn't, then it's not healing. The component has to be from life!"

- Dr. Sebi

His real name is Alfredo Darrington Bowman; he was a Honduran herbalist healer. He did his herbal practice in the United States during the late 20th and 21st centuries. Dr. Sebi claimed that he could cure all diseases with his vegan herbs and diet, including AIDS. He also said that H.I.V. was not the cause of AIDS. Sebi proved that he could cure AIDS, as he had several patients who came with the illness and were cured of AIDS after using Sebi's herbs.

Bowman had a treatment center in a village near La Ceiba, Honduras, before moving his herbal practice to Los Angeles and New York City. The Honduras native had several celebrities as his clients. Some of them include Eddie Murphy, Steven Seagal, Lisa Lopez, and Michael Jackson. Bowman did not attend any medical training; the expertise he received was the herbal knowledge passed to him by his grandmother. So, you'll never find a doctor's license hanging on his wall, but in place of this, he had a herbal training certificate.

That made licensed medical practitioners consider Sebi as a quack. He did not agree with Western medicine and practice. Bowman's dissatisfaction with Western medicine originated when doctors failed after several attempts to cure him of diabetes, asthma, visual impairment, and impotence. He traveled to Mexico to visit a herbalist name Alfredo Cortez, where he finally had the cure he wanted. He cured him of his diseases, something that Western medicine failed to do.

After his recovery, Sebi dedicated his life to herbal practice and began his practice in Honduras. He cured several patients of all kinds of sickness, so the locals in Honduras started calling him Dr. Sebi because he cured diseases they felt only doctors could cure. Dr. Sebi developed his treatment and called it the "African Bio-Electric Cell Food Therapy," which he claimed could cure various diseases, including the AIDS, cancer, mental illness, and chronic conditions.

As earlier mentioned, Bowman started his treatment center in Honduras and called this center the "USHA Research Institute" located in Usha's. He started marketing his product to the United States before he relocated to New York. Relocating to the United States was not an easy one for him. He was faced with legal opposition to his herbal practice and therapeutic claims. Most of these legal oppositions started crawling in when he claimed his herbal supplements could Cure Aids and because he had no medical license.

During the early 1980s, AIDS had just been recognized as a disease that started as a confined epidemic in the United States, having several cases in New York, Los Angeles, and other cities. Bowman opposed medical practitioners, saying H.I.V. was not the curse of Aids and used his herbal products to cure people. In May 2016, He was arrested for money laundering, where he spent weeks in detention, which lead to him contracting pneumonia. On August 6, 2016, he died on his way to hospital D'Antoni still in police custody.

CHAPTER ONE

HERBS AND THE HEALING PROCESS

Before the birth of Western pharmacological medicine, several individuals resorted to using herbal or traditional medicines, which are of plant origin, to treat disease. Nevertheless, Western medicine practice believes its methods are the best, which has been proven otherwise. Research has shown that close to 60% of pharmaceutical drugs are generated from plants, whether directly or indirectly.

Before the socioeconomic marginalization of the world that coerced people from third world countries to believe that western medicine was the only remedy for diseases, indigenous people understood the functions of various plants in their environment and used them to reverse different diseases. Medicinal herbs are quite different from plant foods or food herbs because they contain a higher concentration of Phytonutrients, which plays a major role in traditional medicine.

Medicinal herbs are also bitter compared to food herbs. Western medicine makes these plants or herbs taste better by adding some clinical additives to improve the taste. The healing process of the body is natural, being that the body is made up of cells, tissues, and organs that are meant to self-correct and heal themselves. The body system is designed to repair worn-out cells, resist and kill disease, and destroy damaged body cells. Throughout the lifespan of any human, the body is continuously building new cells, replacing old ones, and replicating others.

Proteins

The body's healing process starts with getting rid of foods or diets that introduce pathogens and toxins into the system. These toxins are responsible for mucus buildup, which the herbalist Dr. Sebi believes is the cause of diseases.

Recent research carried out by the World Health Organization (WHO) revealed that processed meat or red meats are carcinogenic to humans. These scientific studies carried out by the said medical practitioners have proven that animal fat and animal protein increase the risk of diabetes, cancer, heart disease, and other lethal chronic diseases. This is one reason why Dr. Sebi wants humans to implore the natural healing process of alkaline non-hybrid plants, which he believes is the foundation for health and Healing.

Diets that contain toxin and acid causes the body to be prone to attacks like inflammatory reactions, leading to chronic inflammation. Acute inflammation is a natural process that helps the body fight against infections or diseases and also extends to repair damaged tissues and cells in the body. But when it becomes excessive, the natural process, which is intended to fight or resist diseases, starts to compromise the body system itself by attacking healthy cells, leading to different diseases.

This disorderliness leads to the overproduction of mucus by the mucous membrane, which extends to compromise healthy organs. Dr. Sebi says that we have to start eliminating such foods from our diets to attain the natural healing process, including processed foods, meat, dairy, and other unnatural acidic plant foods.

Dr. Sebi did not include or promote "animal protein" in his vegan diets because he believes it interferes with the natural healing process. Nitrogen is known to be the building blocks of enzymes and muscle. These building blocks are derived from the assimilation of nitrogenous compounds. Western medicine and practitioners have conditioned people into thinking that animal-based proteins, like meat, are essential, which Dr. Sebi opposes. In 1914, a study was carried out on infant rats and showed that infant rats grew faster when consumed animal protein. It led to the meat industry's potent campaign that animal protein was better than vegetable protein, an idea which intention was to promote the consumption of a Western diet but can be traced to chronic diseases.

The Meat Industry Campaign portrayed plant protein as an incomplete protein, meaning that vegetable or plant protein did not contain the body's nine essential amino acids. Nevertheless, the 1914 study was acknowledged to be incorrect by some organizations like the American

Heart Organization, and they regarded vegetable protein as a complete protein. This didn't matter much because the meat industry had influenced health organizations to promote meat protein over vegetable sources, hence the status quo of chronic diseases in our world today.

In recent research carried out by the World Health Organization, animal protein consumption has been linked to cancerous cells' accelerated growth if these proteins are consumed excessively (10% more) of the daily calories. On the other hand, vegetable sources regulate and support human growth naturally without promoting harmful organisms.

CHAPTER TWO

WHAT ARE DR.SEBI APPROVED HERBS?

"If Nature didn't make it, don't take it"

- Dr. Sebi.

I created this chapter to help anyone who wants their body to heal and revitalized using Nature's greatest gift, "Herbs." Dr. Sebi, until his death, lived his life as a biochemist, pathologist, and naturalist. During his lifetime of research, he identified herbs with an active healing ingredient in places like North and South America, and Central America, the Caribbean, and Africa. He used these herbs to establish a unique methodology and system that can set up real Healing on the human body. All the herbs he introduced and recommended were entrenched in his over 30 years of experience.

The list of food he considered toxic includes most synthetic and processed food like fried food, iodized salt, alcohol (western diet), and sugar. Based on his belief and recommendation, substituting most of the synthesized food items that are toxic to health with food like raw nuts, grains, green vegetables, fruits, and grains will energize the body's immune system and increase the healing potentials of the body. What made Dr.Sebi stand out is that most of his methodology was centered on Alkaline Foods and Medicinal Herbs.

The table below contains some of the doctor Sebi's approved Herbs. All the herbs mentioned in the table are products that support his work:

Anamu/Guinea Hen Weed	whole Herb
Arnica	Flower, Root
Basil	Leaf, Essential Oil
Bladderwrack	Whole Herb
Bay leaves	Leaf
Bugleweed	Aerial parts
Blue Vervain	Leaf, Flower
Burdock	Root
Cancansa/Cansasa/Red Willow Bark	Bark

Catnip	Aerial Parts
Cannabis (Marijuana/ Hemp)	Flower, leaf, seed, stem

Cardo Santo/Blessed Thistle/Holy Thistle	Aerial Part
Capadula	Bark, Root
Cayenne/African Bird Pepper	Fruit
Cascara Sagrada/Sacred Bark	Bark
Centaury/Star Thistle/ Knapweed	Flowering Aerial Parts
Chaparro Amargo	Leaf, Branch
Chickweed	Whole Herb
Chamomile	Flower, Leaf
Clove	Undeveloped Flower Bud
Cocolmeca	Root
Condurango	Vine, Bark
Contribo/Birthwort	Root, Aerial Part
Cuachalalate	Bark
Cordoncillo Negro	Bark

Elderberry	Berry, Flower
Drago/Dracaena Draco/ Dragon Tree	Leaf, Bark
Dandelion	Root, Leaf (Mainly root used as medicine)
Feverfew/Santa Maria	Whole Plant, Root, Flowering & Fruiting
Fennel	Seed
Eyebright	Aerial Parts
Eucalyptus	Leaf
Flor de Manita/Hand Flower Tree	Flower
Guaco/Mikania	Root
Ginger	Root
Hoodia Gordonii/ Kalahari Cactus	The fleshy part of the stem
Governadora/Chaparral	Leaf/Flower
Hombre Grande/ Quassia/Bitter Wood	Bark

Henrique/Werke	Root
Hortensia/Hydrangea	Dried Rhizome, Root

Hortensia/Hydrangea	Dried Rhizome, Root
Kalawalla	Rhizome, Frond, Leaf
Kinkeliba/Seh Haw	Leaf, Root, and Bark
Linden	Flower
Lily of the Valley	Flower
Lemon Verbena	Leaves, Flowering Top
Lavender	Flower, Leaves
Lupulo/Hops	Flower
Locust	Bark
Lirio/Lily	Flower, Bulb, Leaf
Eucalyptus	Leaf
Hortensia/Hydrangea	Dried Rhizome, Root

Lirio/Lily	Flower, Bulb, Leaf
Manzo	Root, Rhizome, Leaf
Lily of the Valley	Flower
Arnica	Root, Flower
Lavender	Flower, Leaves
Eyebright	Aerial Parts

Santa Maria/Sage	Leaf
Condurango	Vine, Bark
Linden	Flower
Tila/Linden	Flower
Palo Mulato	Bark
Lupulo/Hops	Flower
Centaury/Star Thistle/ Knapweed	Flowering Aerial Parts
Red Clover	Flower

Chamomile	Flower, Leaf
Salsify/Goatsbeard/ Oyster Plant	Root, Leaves, Flower, Seed, Young Stem
Bay leaves	Leaf
Basil	Leaf, Essential Oil
Clove	Undeveloped Flower Bud
Fennel	Seed
Ginger	Root
Cayenne/African Bird Pepper	Fruit
Purslane/Verdolaga	Leaf, Young Shoot, Stem
Soursop	Leaf
Red Raspberry	Leaf
Cuachalalate	Bark
Milk Thistle	Seed
Shepherd's Purse	Whole Herb
Capadula	Bark, Root

Sensitive/Shameplant/ Dead and Wake	Dried Whole Plant, Root, Leaf, Seed
Locust	Bark
Yohimbe	Bark
Myrrh	Resin
Hombre Grande/ Quassia/Bitter Wood	Bark
Oak Bark / Encino	Bark

What is Dr. Sebi Diet?

Sebi claimed that disease results from acidity and mucus in the body and argued that diseases have little or no chance of survival in an alkaline environment. **Here is a brief overview of the foods recommended in his nutritional guide:**

Food	Examples

Vegetables:	Tomatillo, turnip greens, zucchini, watercress, purslane, wild arugula, dandelion greens, garbanzo beans, izote, kale, lettuce (all except Iceberg), mushrooms (all except shiitake), nopales, okra, olives, Amaranth greens, avocado, bell peppers, chayote, cucumber, dandelion greens, garbanzo beans, izote, kale.
Fruits	peaches, pears, plums, prickly pears, prunes, raisins (seeded), soft jelly coconuts, soursops, tamarind, cantaloupe, cherries, currants, dates, figs, grapes (seeded), limes, Apples, bananas, berries (all varieties, no cranberries),

Natural herbal teas	Burdock, chamomile, ginger, raspberry, tila, elderberry, fennel,
Grains	kamut, quinoa, Amaranth, fonio, rye, spelled, tef, wild rice

Nuts and seeds	Hemp seeds, raw sesame seeds, raw sesame "tahini" butter, walnuts, brazil nuts
Oils	Olive oil (do not cook), coconut oil (do not cook), grapeseed oil, sesame oil, hempseed oil, avocado oil
Seasonings and spices	Basil, bay leaf, cloves, dill, oregano, savory, sweet basil, tarragon, thyme, achiote, cayenne, onion powder, habanero, sage, pure sea salt, powdered, granulated seaweed, pure agave syrup, date sugar

Some other rules of Sebi's nutritional guide include:

When you eat any of the food listed on Dr. Sebi's Nutritional Guide

- You must drink one gallon of natural spring water daily.

- Products from animals are strictly prohibited; these include fish, hybrid, and diary.

- Alcohol is not allowed.

- Microwaves are prohibited

- No seedless or canned fruit is allowed.

- You must avoid wheat and only consume the natural growing grains listed.

CHAPTER THREE

HEALING HERBS AND THEIR COMMON USES

"All that man needs for health and healing has been provided by God in nature; the challenge of science is to find it."

- Paracelsus (1493- 1541)

If you're not growing medical herbs, this is a great year to start; with an overwhelmed medical system, it means that things that you can normally get help with maybe less accessible. As someone who wants to help out the medical system and care for people who are most in need, this is a great time to learn how to treat the most common illness or health issue at home; taking this fruitful step will help lessen the excessive demand place on our medical system.

And using herbs is one of the best ways to get around.

One of the major questions I'm asked most often is which herb should I grow in my garden; the answer here is simple. I encourage growing herbs that remedy most of the health problems you regularly have in your family. When I encourage people to stick to herbs that work best for them. Around 50% -60% of people don't even know where to start, which is one of the reasons why I decided to include this chapter. Most of the herbs I mentioned below cover basic illness, so let's dive into these natural healers without further ado.

Chaparral

Chaparral (Larrea Tridentecte):

Has incredible antioxidant power. Most native Americans used this herb to treat various respiratory illnesses and other health conditions like snake bite, chickenpox, and arthritis pain. The herb has powerful antioxidant properties, which makes it perfect it comes to treating the liver, improving immunity, cleansing the blood, and improving overall wellbeing. You can also use this to treat digestive problems like cramps and gas and other respiratory conditions. It serves as an antitumor agent; it contains a nor-dihihydroguairetic (NDGA), a compound that inhibits the energy generated by cancerous cells. It limits the growth of cell proliferation, which can damage the D.N.A.

Chaparral is also used as a mouthwash, irrespective of the awful odor and flavor it gives off. It can further eliminate bacteria that cause tooth decay. The strong antimicrobial and anti-fungal properties made it perfect for treating parasitic paste that lives in the body. It is also used to treat burns; the resin plays a major role in treating skin burns. A cup of Chaparral tea will help you reduce respiratory difficulties; for example, the effects of bronchitis and colds can be alleviated with a cup of tea. This herb is a major expectorant that can help boost your airways' performance and help clear off excessive mucus from the throat. Chaparral has a high percentage of antiinflammatory properties and will help relieve pains from conditions like arthritis.

It can also remedy itch that results from chickenpox, heal bruises, soothe rashes on the skin, heal wounds, and prevent diseases. The herb is also advantageous to fellows suffering from psoriasis and Eczema. Using chaparral as a tea or capsules will remedy digestive problems and combat cancer. To this effect, the herb is suggested by most herbal practitioners once signs of cancer are identified in the kidney, liver, or belly. Additionally, studies show that the herb might inhibit the development of tumors. This herb will help to:

- Remedy digestive issues

- Combat cancer

- Perfect for Eczema and psoriasis

- Help with kidney, liver, and belly issues.

- Serves as an antitumor

  agent

- Use as a mouth wash

Chamomile

Chamomile is known to boost the immune system and reduce muscle spasms, stress, menstrual pain, soothes cold, ache, treat cuts, skin conditions, stomachache, insomnia, and brighten the skin. The herb is known for its unique properties that help to elevate insomnia and boost sleep. It contains an antioxidant called Apigenin; this compound is known to bind some receptors in the brain, promoting sleep and relaxations. Chamomile can relieve stomach ulcers by inhibiting the bacteria that leads to ulcers and reducing the stomach walls' acidity.

Test-tube research shows that Apigenin can combat cancer cells, especially the cancer of the breast, skin, uterus, digestive tract, and prostate. The anti-inflammatory characteristics can help prevent damage to pancreatic cells. These cells are responsible for producing hormones called insulin, which help regulate blood sugar levels. The herb also reduces body cholesterol and blood pressure, which are the major marker for heart disease. This herb will help you to:

- Reduce cholesterol

- Reduce blood pressure

- Lower blood sugar

- Combat cancer

- Promote sleep and relaxation

Chickweed

Chickweed tea is an essential remedy for weight loss. This herb is used among herbal practitioners as a hunger suppressant. Chickweed is known to soothe hunger and relieve other minor irritation within the digestive tract. Once you have a combination of this herb with other medical herbs, it becomes super active.

The herb can also flush the body system and reduce excess water by helping you urinate often. It also serves as a remedy for constipation and bowel issues. The Diuretic effect helps to flush off excess water from the body system by increasing urine. Demulcent creates a soothing film on the mucous membrane; this helps the body to relieve minor pain and inflammation on the membrane. It can be used for:

- Stomach

- Bowel issues

- Constipation

- Blood disorder

- Lung disease

- Asthma

- Scurvy

- Psoriasis

- Itching

- Muscle and joint pain.

The herb can be taken directly or applied on the skin's surface in terms of skin conditions, like abscesses, ulcers, and boils.

Cleavers

Most herbal practitioners regard this herb as a valuable lymphatic tonic and diuretic. The lymph system is a body mechanism that helps wash toxins stored in the bloodstream and help the kidneys and the liver. This action sets the herb apart as one of the best remedies for treating health conditions like arthritis and psoriasis. They are also known as a reliable diuretic that can also treat urinary infections and help eliminate urinary stone and gravel.

Cloves

This herb is used to:

- Stop bad breath

- Treat nausea and vomiting.

- Relieves joint pain,

- Soothes toothpaste

- Improves digestion

- Improve respiratory condition

- Eases earaches

- Fight stress

- Cures aches

Cocolmeca

Cocolmeca (Smilax, smilax reguli, Smilax aristolochiifolia, Jamaican sarsaparilla cocolmeca bark, cuculmeca) are known for their antiulcer, anticancer, diuretic, diaphoretic, and antioxidant properties. Cocolmeca belongs to the smilax genus, and it is known to bind with toxins and boost body health. This herb is used traditionally to treat different skin conditions like:

- Leprosy

- Psoriasis

- Joint pain

- Cold

- Sexual impotence

- Rheumatoid arthritis

Contribo

Contribo (Birthwort, Hierba del Indio Aristolochia, Aristolochia Grandiflora, duck flower, Alcatraz). The Contribo herb is used to remedy both edema and arthritis, to boost the immune system. It is also used as a treatment to increase the overall production of white blood cells in order to eliminate bladder stones, gout, uterine complaints, kill parasites, kidney ailments. It is also well-known for treating snake bite. However, this herb is not recommended commercially due to the poisonous content.

Caution: not recommended for nursing, and pregnant women are advised to stay away from this herb due to its toxic effect on the kidney. If they are required to do so for some reason, it should be under the supervision of a herbalist or an expert.

Dimiana

Dimiana (Damiana leaf, Turnera diffusa, damiana aphrodisiac, turnera, tunera aphrodisiac, damiana herb) is known for its anti-anxiety anti-aromatase property. It is recommended for both men and women to boost sexual drive and strengthen their sexual organs. It contains an anti-aromatase property that blocks androstenedione and estrone conversion to estrogen. Damiana herbs are also used to control other forms of illness that result from estrogen-like fibroids and breast cancer. Damiana boosts the quality of oxygen that is transferred to the genitals, which improves libido. It is also used to remedy PTSD, depression, nervousness, and relieve the anxiety that results from sexual dysfunction. The herb can also increase intestinal traction and remedy constipation. It is very rich in vitamins and minerals; the herb is used to:

- Reduce flashes that are related to menopause

- Treat vaginal dryness

- Treat headache

- Enhance mood

- Increase physical and mental stamina

- Promote weight loss

- Support testosterone level in men

- Balance estrogen in women

Dandelion root

Dandelion helps to maintain healthy bones since it is very rich in calcium. The root can also be used as a substitute for coffee. Dandelions can be used to treat hemorrhaging in the liver, intestinal gas, gallstones, upset stomach, loss of appetite, bruises, Eczema, and muscle aches. The herb is known to increase urine production and act as a laxative that helps boost movement in the bowel. For those who use it to treat viral infection and cancer, it rich elements make it a skin toner, digestive tonic, and blood tonic. Calcium is one of the major elements found in the body. It is needed in the body for strong teeth and bones. It helps nerve transmission, hormone secretion, blood clotting, and muscle contraction.

Eating green dandelion or drinking it as tea can help avoid muscle tension, high blood pressure and tooth decay, and other health condition that are likely to occur due to calcium deficiency. The herb is rich in Vitamin K, one of the major vitamins essential for blood clotting and mineralization; it is also known to build the bones! Vitamin K also increases body metabolism and the function of the brain. It cleans the liver, boosts the skin and fights diabetes. This super herb contains high levels of antioxidants, especially rich in vitamin A. It helps prevent urinary tract infection and serves as a diuretic. Dandelion Root can be used to relieve the following disorders:

- Eczema

- Muscle aches

- Liver hemorrhage

- Intestinal gas

- Upset in the stomach

- Gallstones

- Urinary disorders

- Diabetes

- Ache

- Jaundice

- Anemia

- Cancer

Anamu

Anamu (Mucura, Apacina Guinea Henweed) is one of the most interesting plants I have seen throughout my carrier; the plant has active properties that can be used to combat cancerous cells. It fights infections demonstrates a broad-spectrum antimicrobial effect against a wide range of viruses, fungi, bacteria, and yeast. The yeast compound can kill or inhibits the growth of germs. This herb is widely used to treat infections, and it is known to also relieve pain; this means it can be used to remedy the pain -generated from rheumatism and arthritis. The herb is also validated by clinical research that it serves as an anti-inflammatory and pain-relieving effect.

When Anamu extract is topically applied directly to the skin, it relieves pain and inflammation. Anamu lower blood sugar, and records have it that it used in Cuba to remedy diabetes. The herb can also lead to contraction of the uterus, which, as a result, can lead to miscarriages or abortions; this is why it is not recommended for pregnant women. The herb has a low concentration of blood thinner known as Coumadin. People suffering from bleeding disorders like hemophilia should seek the attention of an expert before using the herb. I recommend using an originally grown Anamu herb that is free from insecticides, herbicides, and other forms of chemical pollution.

To create the magic: use one heaped tablespoon of Anamu plant and add it to 1liter of hot water. Allow it to dissolve properly and take it as a tea; I recommend doing this on an empty stomach and sticking to an average dose of four-ounce twice a day. Anamu can be used to:

- Lower blood sugar

- Use as a broad-spectrum antimicrobial

Arnica

Arnica (Radix Ptamica Montana, Arnica Montana, mountain tobacco, arnica flowers) is an antiseptic and anti-inflammatory herb primarily used to reduce pain and treat external wounds due to its effectiveness in terms of regeneration of tissues. Arnica can be applied externally as body cream and used to treat sprains, arthritis, headaches, and bruise. Arnica infusions have enough antiseptic properties; this feature makes them effective when used to clean wounds, boils, and abscesses.

Dr. Sebi uses this herb as one of his uterine wash compounds. It is used externally on the skin to heal and soothe bruises and relieve irritation resulting from arthritis, trauma, cartilage, and muscle pain. When used for arthritis, I recommend using it as a topical cream over the affected area. This herb can help with:

- Arthritis

- Relieve pain

- Relieve headaches

- Pain from bruises

- Treat sprains

- Boils

- Abscesses

Ashwagandha

This adaptogenic herb is prevalent in Ayurveda medicine and has been used by herbalists for the past 25,000 years. I firmly believe you've seen the herb or read about it before; it's one of the most popular and commonly used adaptogen herbs. It is known for modulating the thyroid, its neuroprotective anti-depressant, and anti-anxiety properties are associated as some of the benefits. In India, the herb is called the "Strength of the Stallion" and is traditionally used to boost the immune system after illness. It can as well increase your body's stamina and help you to relieve stress.

It is also used as a stress-protective agent, which is one reason it is widely known. It helps the body maintain homeostasis during physical and emotional stress. What's more? The herb shows remarkable results in terms of lowering cortisol and striking a balance in thyroid hormones. Additionally, it is also used to prevent degenerative diseases and mood disorder. This herb is used to:

- Lower cortisol

- Balance the thyroid hormone

- Prevent degenerative diseases

- Enhance mood

- Maintain homeostasis

- Anti-stress

- Boost immune system

Eyebright

Eyebright (Euphrasia rostkoviana, Euphrasia Officinalis) this herb has plenty of antiseptic and anti-inflammatory and it's perfect when used as an eyewash to soothe mucous and treat inflammation. It serves as an antimicrobial, and it is used to treat blepharitis and conjunctivitis. It also serves as astringent use to treat wounds and inflammation of the skin. Most herbal practitioners have repeatedly used it in treating upper respiratory tract infections like hay fever and sinusitis. The herb can minimize discomfort due to its phytonutrients. It contains antiinflammatory action, soothing inflamed and tired eyes, which also helps reduce secretions and relieve the mucous membrane's inflammation, especially in patients suffering from blepharitis and conjunctivitis.

Eyebright is effective when used on styes due to catteic acid, which is known to combat infection. It allows the eye to absorb minerals, zinc selenium, and copper; this element help protect against cataract, one of the major cause of blindness. Eyebright contains natural astringent tannins, which are known to reduce the formation of mucus and catarrh. Tannins' element helps to tighten the mucous membrane, while the flavonoid content in the herb gives off instant relief from allergies like cold, cough and other forms of chest infection. This herb will help you combat infections like:

- Blepharitis

- Conjunctivitis

- Serves as anti-inflammatory

- Treat wounds and skin inflammations.

Bladderwrack

Bladderwrack (Fucus, Fucus Vesiculosus) this herb is used for its medicinal benefits for centuries now. One of its major use is to stimulate the thyroid gland and help treat cellulite and obesity. The herb contains a significant amount of iodine, which helps to boost the performance of the thyroid. It helps relieve symptoms of rheumatoid and rheumatism arthritis and can also be used externally and internally. This herb is recommended because of its iodine content, which is known to boost the body's metabolism. Over time, it has been repeatedly used to treat oversize and under-active thyroid, iodine deficiency, cellulite, and obesity. Bladderwrack is rich in calcium, potassium, magnesium, and other trace elements essential to the body.

The anti-estrogenic effect helps reduce the risk of estrogen-dependent disease. Bladderwrack helps to reduce body cholesterol levels and also supports weight loss. It contains phytonutrients and mucopolysaccharides that inhibit skin enzymes that break the skin, improve skin elasticity, and minimize skin thickness. The herb has rich anti-candida antitumor and antibacterial properties. Bladderwrack is a natural iodine supplement; the herb can be used for:

- Blood cleansing

- Heartburn

- Digestive disorder

- Bronchitis

- Constipation

- Emphysema

- Urinary tract infection

- Anxiety

- Increase blood circulations

- Protect the skin

- Strengthen the heart

Devil's Claw root

This plant is most common in South Africa, and native herbalists long use it due to its inflammatory response, tonify digestion, and pain management effect. And due to its medicinal benefits, the plant was later grown in Europe back in the late 1800s. This plant helps to Harden the walls of the arteries (atherosclerosis)

- Gout

- Muscle pain (myalgia)

- Back pain

- Arthritis

- Fibromyalgia

- Tendonitis

- Gastrointestinal (G.I.) upset

- Fever

- Heartburn

- Migraine headache

- Chest pain

Dr.Sebi recommends a daily dose is of 600–2,610 mg.

Dr.Sebi's medicinal herbs were designed for anyone aiming to naturally cure or prevent disease restoring their body's natural balance and improve overall health without relying on conventional Western medicine. These herbal treatments combined with Dr.Sebi's Alkaline Plant based diet are a great way of ensuring that there's no space for disease in your body.

Amber Florey

BOOK 2

Dr. SEBI

Alkaline Diet and herbal detox: How to naturally prevent and cure diabetes, high blood pressure and heart disease: includes recipes and herb preparation advice

AMBER FLOREY

INTRODUCTION

WHO IS DR. SEBI

It goes without saying that diet plays an important role in the life of every individual. It goes a long way in determining the quality of life that individuals enjoy. For instance, a good diet with adequate quality and quantity will result in better health and well-being. On the other hand, a poor diet with inconsistency in quality and quantity will only harm the body.

Various types of diseases may emerge, ranging from mucus and discharge to more serous chronic diseases. The good news is that this is there is something we can do about it. By maintaining a proper diet, it is possible to improve the situation and maintain a high quality of life.

This was the belief of Alfredo Bowman, now popularly known as Dr. Sebi.

ALFREDO DARRINGTON BOWMAN

Alfredo Darrington Bowman was born on the 26th of November, 1993. He was born in Honduras. A man of African descent, Dr. Sebi took pride in his roots. He referred to himself as an "African in Honduras" rather than succumbing to the "African Honduras" tag.

His early life provided him access to herbal healing as he learned the rudiments from his grandmother. Later, he proceeded to expand the horizon of herbal healing to various illnesses. However, just before that, Dr. Sebi needed the spur of ineffective western medical care when treating his illness.

He suffered from a wide range of illnesses like asthma, impotence, visual impairment, and diabetes. Then, after various trials with western medical practices, he found these procedures quite ineffective in his case. So, he proceeded to visit a Mexican herbalist named Alfredo Cortez. According to Dr. Sebi, the herbalist confirmed that his death was imminent. However, the herbalist was able to heal himself completely.

Following this, Dr. Sebi returned to Honduras, where he began his healing practice. He based his treatment on herbs. He then developed the "African Bio-Electric Cell Food Therapy" and claimed that this approach could cure various diseases, including AIDS and cancer.

According to Dr. Sebi, his procedure involved cleansing the body of excess mucus. He thought that every disease could be traced back to the compromise of the mucus membrane. So, by cleansing the body of this excess mucus, the body can be in a much better condition. For instance, according to him, the accumulation of mucus in the joint is what results in arthritis. In the same vein, the accumulation of mucus in the bronchus is what causes bronchitis. Now, by clearing this mucus, this condition can disappear.

As such, Dr. Sebi pushed for an alkaline diet to ensure that the body remains in top condition. Various reports have established that his diet was effective as he used his approach to reverse a wide range of incurable ailments. He applied his approach to a wide range of conditions such as blindness, and mental illness, among others.

Alfredo Darrington Bowman, popularly known as Dr. Sebi, died on the 6th of August, 2016, from Pneumonia related complications. Regardless, he left a legacy that advocated the use of an alkaline diet to achieve wellness.

CHAPTER ONE
ALKALINE VS. ACIDIC FOODS

Introduction

A huge part of healthy living is an alkalized body. This helps to ensure that the body remains in a state where metabolism occurs effectively, and the body retains its structural integrity. However, one way of achieving this is finding a balance between the acidic and alkaline levels within the body.

According to recent studies, every healthy body must possess an 80 percent alkaline and a 20 percent acidic level. Anything disrupting this balance will result in an imbalance of the body system. This will then give room for the emergence of a wide range of diseases within the body.

The most consumed foods in our modern society are high acidic and low alkaline. Unfortunately for us, to ensure the proper functioning of the body, an important element is that individuals must increase the intake of alkaline-based foods compared to acidic foods. Everyone must consume three times more alkaline-based food than acidic food.

For instance, proteins, sugars, processed foods, cereals, and junk foods are all high in acidic content rather than alkaline. Yet, that is what most individuals consume the most. On the other hand, alkaline foods like vegetables and fruits are rarely consumed. At best, individuals consume them in smaller quantities, thus tipping the scale in favor of acidic food.

Since there is not enough alkaline to neutralize the ever-increasing intake of acidic foods, the body records higher acidity. This is not an ideal state for your body to be because it attracts a wide range of illnesses while weakening the immune system that should be responsible for defending you.

Understanding the body's alkaline/acid balance

It is important to note that this is restricted to the body's pH level when we talk about the body's alkaline/acid balance. It is necessary to keep this in mind because it is easy to confuse this with stomach acid.

In the former's case, this involves the pH level of the body fluids, tissues, and cells. Now, these various parts and constituents of the body do not in any way, benefit from a high acidic level. Instead, they are harmed by a high acidic level as it affects their normal functioning and performance. For instance, high acidity in these various bodies constitutes the major cause of high blood pressure in humans.

However, in the latter case, this is limited to the stomach's pH level, which is naturally and always acidic. So, your food intake does not affect your stomach's acidity as it needs this acidity to engage in proper digestion of ingested food substances.

Distinguishing between acidic and alkaline foods

One thing that you might find difficult to do is to distinguish between acidic foods and alkaline foods. Let's just look at one example: most people regard lemons as acidic foods when, in fact, the reality is far from this. Without a doubt, lemon contains citric acid. However, this does not translate to the fact that they are acidic when it comes to your body's pH level. In fact, lemons have an alkalizing effect on your body. This is also the same with various fruits like apple cider vinegar, which people confuse as acidic when they are, in fact, alkaline food types.

Typically, alkaline foods are food options that possess high mineral constituents but low acid content. On the other hand, acidic foods are those with sugar constituents. Sugar typically ferments inside the human body and transforms into acid.

So, when we talk about acidic food, we mean that you need to avoid food substances that are high in sugar contents. They pose significant harm to man's health. On the other hand, when you talk about alkaline foods, we mean high mineral content, which flushes out toxins from your body.

So, here are top examples of alkaline-rich fruits.

- Lemons
- Tomatoes
- Coconut
- Avocado
- Pomegranate
- Grapefruit
- Limes

Also, examples of alkaline-rich veggies include:

- Cabbage
- Broccoli
- Celery
- Kale
- Spinach
- Parsley
- Alfalfa Sprouts
- Garlic
- Endive

Problems With a high acidic food intake

Further, note that the concentration of highly acidic food comes with various side effects in your body. These side effects cut across the following areas.

1. UNHEALTHY SKIN, HAIR, AND NAILS

One effect of a high concentration of acid within the body is unhealthy skin, hair, and nails. Precisely, when it comes to the nails, they become so weak and thin. In turn, they break easily and upon the slightest contact.

In the same vein, individuals with a high acidic level in their cells and tissues will experience extremely dry skin. They will also suffer from a pale face. This can also extend to the emergence of cracks around the lips.

When it comes to hair, it is usually dull with split ends as it begins to fall out.

2. DIGESTIVE ISSUES

Another issue that may arise in the event of a high acidic level in the body is digestive issues. This involves situations where the body has a problem carrying out the digestive process effectively. This will cut across issues like excess stomach acid, gastritis, saliva acidic, ulcers, and acid reflux. Note that due to the relevance of digestion within the body, this situation can go a long way to harm the body.

3. MOUTH AND TEETH ISSUES

Another problem that may arise in high acidic content within the body is issues with the mouth and teeth. Typically, these issues will bring a wide range of discomfort to the mouth.

Vivid examples of results of this high acidic content within the mouth include tooth sensitivity. Even more, the tooth may display a tendency or susceptibility to chipping and cracking.

Other issues include mouth ulcers, which will make talking and swelling more difficult. Furthermore, such individuals can experience tooth nerve discomfort and pain in addition to having sensitive gums.

There is also the case of getting a loose tooth or suffering from infections to the tonsils and throat.

4. GENERAL BODY, EYES, AND HEAD

Individuals who consume a high level of acidic foods may also suffer general body pain and may suffer from specific discomfort in the eye and head area.

When it comes to the general body, they may be more susceptible to infections. Also, experiencing a lower body temperature than previously recorded. Worse, they might suffer from headaches, both mild and severe.

They might also suffer from leg cramps, spasms, conjunctivitis. All this will leave the body and eye feeling less comfortable than it should be. There have been cases of corneas and eyelids inflammation associated with high intake of food with acidic contents.

5. EMOTIONS AND NERVES

The regular consumption of food high in acidic contents can lead to complications and issues with the nervous system and control over emotions. In some cases, it will lead to a feeling of constant fatigue buy the patient. In the same vein, there may be a case of excessive nervousness when it comes to such a person. They also are in a situation where they feel depressed and unable to connect with emotions of enthusiasm and joy.

Benefits of high alkaline food intake

Finding a balance between your intake of acidic food and alkaline food intake can be quite challenging. However, it remains an endeavor that you must continue to invest your time and resources in. This is thanks to the wide range of advantages that it comes with.

These advantages are as follows:

1. ANTI-AGING

The alkaline diet is also known to many as the antiaging diet! Who doesn't want to look younger? Various reports and studies associate the occurrence of aging with the emergence of gray hair and wrinkles. However, this is merely the result of a series of processes that occur internally. The aging process takes place within the body where it is impossible to see it.

The process of aging is accelerated by the increased presence of acid within the body. If your body maintains the necessary alkaline balance, you can look youthful as you slow down the aging process.

By sticking to an alkaline diet your skin will definitely see an improvement: your collagen production will increase, inflammation is reduced and your skin will become less dry and have a more natural glow to it.

2. IMPROVED JOINT HEALTH

People with a higher intake of acidic diet are more likely to suffer from arthritis. This is because the increased acidic content increases the rate at which the bones and cartilage degenerate. Even worse, it reduces one's motion.

On the other hand, the right intake of an alkaline-based diet reduces the acidic contents within the body. In turn, you will not have to worry about issues related to poor joints. This is because it reduces the likelihood of inflammation by increasing circulation in the joint. In turn, one can expedite better overall joint health.

3. IMPROVED IMMUNITY

This is another significant function that adequate intake of alkaline-based food plays in the body. This is significant because your immune system is one of the most vital components if you are looking to maintain good health.

Precisely, it is responsible for providing your body with antibodies that combat invaders and microorganisms.

This process occurs naturally through what we call phagocytosis. This process functions to expel these foreign entities from your body circulation. For this process to work effectively, it requires a balance of the body's pH levels. Too much acidity will ruin this process, causing more damage.

However, you can be sure that this natural process will work correctly with the right alkaline balance allowing your immune system will function more effectively.

4. IMPROVED MENTAL CLARITY

Another advantage that comes with the right alkaline balance is mental clarity. Typically, with aging comes mental decline. However, with increased acidic content intake, there is a reduction in the production of necessary and functioning neurotransmitters. This will then increase the likelihood of mental decline.

Furthermore, various research has established that with increased acidic pH levels comes various neurodegenerative diseases. Fortunately, with increased intake of an alkalinebased diet, you can achieve the necessary balance. This will then ensure the increase in neurotransmitter production and improved mental activity and clarity.

So, you will not need to worry about dementia or Alzheimer's diseases, or any other neurodegenerative disorders. An alkaline-based diet helps you to reduce the likelihood of their emergence.

5. IMPROVED ENERGY ACCESS

Another benefit that accompanies the right intake of alkaline in the body is improved energy. Typically, with

high acidic intake comes increased fatigue and feelings of sluggishness. This is because the metabolic pathways do not function at their best anymore. Rather, they begin to slow down, which emerges as fatigue.

However, with an adequate alkaline-based diet, you can get the right balance. In turn, your body's metabolic process will function at the right level, which allows you to get easy access to energy and remain agile.

6. EASY WEIGHT LOSS

With the accumulation of various toxins in the body, weight loss is sure to become difficult. This will typically be because these toxins begin to get stored in fat thanks to the high acidic level. On the other hand, by getting the right dosage of alkaline-based diet into the body, you can flush out these toxins. This will ensure that there is improved waste elimination from the body and better weight loss.

Acidic vs. alkaline based diet is an area that continues to attract considerable attention. It remains an unavoidable topic thanks to its importance in proper health and wellbeing.

So, every day is the right day to start prioritizing an alkaline based diet. We have listed the basic options above, and we will go into more details in the subsequent chapters. You will also need to avoid various acidic foods such as processed foods, meat products, dairy products, and junk foods, among others.

This way, you can begin your cleansing journey and obtain the best health possible. In the next chapter, we will delve into Dr. Sebi's views on starch consumption and its effect on the human body.

CHAPTER TWO

STARCH BASED DIET LINKED TO DIABETES AND HEART DISEASE

Introduction

A predominant aspect of our diet is the daily intake of starch. Typically, we consume starch in a large proportion each day and perhaps more than any other substance. However, we hardly consider the effect of such a considerable consumption of it in our bodies. The reality is that while most individuals enjoy the sweetening nature of some starch, it is hardly suitable for our body.

It contains some substances and compounds that harm our body in the long run. It is necessary for us to regulate our consumption of starch if we intend to live a healthy life. Noteworthy, this was the belief of Dr. Sebi. He stated that starch contained cyanide, contributing to the destabilization of the body system and brain waves. This notion has been confirmed as western medicine links the high consumption of starches to illnesses like weight gain, heart disease, and type 2 diabetes.

What is starch?

Technically, starch is a subset of carbohydrates and represents the most consumed type of carbohydrate. While it is regarded as a source of energy, it is also classified as complex carbohydrates that consist of multiple sugar molecules.

Although complex carbohydrates are regarded as the healthier option, this is not the case with most of the starch available today. With complex starch, there is a gradual release of sugar to your body. In turn, there is a reduced possibility of a rapid increase in the blood sugar level.

Unfortunately, today, the available starch options are extremely refined. Complex carbohydrates do exist but they can still contribute significantly to a spike in blood sugar levels. This is because most of these food substances have lost most of their fiber and nutrients. They are now empty calories that provide little or no nutritional benefit to your body.

Dr. Sebi on starch

One core idea of Dr. Sebi's Alkaline diet is the negative impacts of starch on the body. According to him, starch represents a non-natural material that contributes to damaging the body. Starch is a binder that works to combine two distinct substances. This imbalance in the molecular structure of starch concentrated foods makes them less desirable for the body.

Furthermore, starch contains various substances that make the alkaline level of the body imbalanced. As discussed in the previous chapter, your body must maintain a balanced alkaline level if it intends to perform optimally.

With too much intake of acidic foods, we destabilize the balance of our body system. In turn, this leaves us susceptible to the accumulation of mucus. As you can now tell, with mucus comes various diseases. Instead, the body needs a higher intake of natural and alkaline substances that maintain our body's metabolism.

Now, this is where starch comes in, and that is what makes it not so desirable for your body. Starch contains a substance that contributes to raising the acidic level of our body. It is examined below.

Cyanide

According to Dr. Sebi, the first constituent of starch that makes it less desirable is cyanide. This is a substance that is quite popular as deadly to the human body. However, this understanding comes primarily from its application to military activities rather than food substances.

Even without delving deeper, it is obvious that a substance applied consistently to military activities cannot be good for the body. This is what individuals now consume when they engage in the daily and arbitrary consumption of starch.

For instance, you can find cyanide traces in food substances like cassava, almonds, and lima beans. No doubt, they consist of a much lower concentration than that applied to military activities. However, considering that these starch foods are consumed in large proportion, it becomes evident that we supply our body with a significant amount of cyanide through starch foods.

Typically, this chemical works by reducing oxygen circulation within the body. This then contributes to the death of cells within the body. It is clear that your cells' death in such a manner is not good for your body. However, this is what comes with cyanide and its consumption through starch concentrated foods.

Eventually, this will lead to various negative body conditions, including damage to the heart, brain, and nerves. One might even experience cases of lung injuries, respiratory issues, low blood pressure, and slow heart rate.

Acrylamide

The presence of acrylamide has also been confirmed in starchy foods. This chemical emerges in various starch concentrated foods like bread and potatoes when they get cooked for an extended period and at high temperatures. For instance, this chemical will emerge in cases of longterm and high-temperature baking, toasting, roasting, grilling, and frying.

Unfortunately, this chemical is also dangerous to your general health. In fact, this chemical can result in the emergence of cancer in the body.

This is not the only condition that the consumption of starch concentrated foods can result in. It can result in a wide range of other conditions like being overweight, having diabetes, and various heart diseases. It can also culminate into the imbalance of the body's alkaline level, which will result in general poor health.

From the preceding, it is clear that although highly preferred as a food item, starch is not healthy for the body. It contributes negatively to your general health. As such, it is not only important, but starch intake must inevitably be controlled to achieve good and healthy living.

Starch and poor nutrient density

Starch also poses other challenges to your health, one of the prominent challenges associated with starch intake is its low nutrients density.

In most cases, various food items that have high starch concentration add little or no nutrients to the body. Precisely, they do not provide any nutrients to your body beyond the addition of carbohydrates and calories. According to Dr. Sebi, this contributes to creating an imbalance in your body's alkaline level.

This is also the case under western medicine, where the rule is to prioritize a balanced diet. That is a diet that provides adequate amounts of all necessary micro and macronutrients. When you assess it from this perspective, starch does not provide an adequate amount of nutrients across the various categories. It merely provides a high concentration of sugar to the body, which is bad news for you.

Also, there is no doubt that some of these starch concentrated foods sometimes contain some positive nutrients. For instance, yucca, plantain, tubers, and potatoes contain some relevant nutrients. However, in the long run, these food items contain considerable starch that far outweighs the acclaimed benefits that come with other nutrients.

According to Dr. Sebi, this becomes less desirable as one can get these other necessary nutrients from less harmful and natural substances. Precisely, various other natural substances provide these other nutrients in better quality and quantity. Even more, they do not attract the health risk that comes with starch concentrated foods. In turn, it makes no sense that anyone should continue to consume starch when there is a much better and healthier alternative.

Food with high starch concentration

Various food substances contain a considerable amount of starch in them. We consider popular examples of such food substances. This way, you can understand what you need to avoid.

1. Cornmeal – 74% Starch Concentration

This is a popular food that most individuals find attractive as a meal. It comes from grinding corn kernels when dry. It then produces s coarse flour that you can consume. Typically, this food is regarded as gluten-free, making it safe for those with celiac diseases.

However, the major challenge with this item is its high starch constituent. With one cup of cornmeal, a whopping 74% is all starch. In turn, the high consumption of cornmeal translates to a significant intake of starch.

2. Rice Krispies Cereal – 72.1% Starch Concentration

Another food item that records a high concentration of starch is the Rice Krispies. This food item comes from crisped rice, a combination of sugar paste and puffed rice. No doubt, while this food item comes with minerals and vitamins, it does not make up for the high starch concentration that it possesses.

This food item is highly processed, and 28 grams of this food contains 20.2 grams of starch, which stands at 72.1%. As such, it would be best if you avoided the consumption of rice Krispies cereal.

3. Pretzels – 71.3% Starch Concentration

Pretzels are one of the most popular snacks that we consume daily. Unfortunately, these snacks do more damage than good. This is thanks to its high starch concentration. Precisely, you get a high 48 grams of starch from every 60 grams of pretzel that you consume.

You will experience fatigue and hunger when you consistently consume this much starch. Even more, it affects the body's ability to regulate its blood sugar level, which is the cause of type 2 diabetes.

4. Flours – 68 to 70% Starch Concentration

Another food item that brings high starch concentration with it is flour. Precisely, depending on the type of flour you take, you can get between 68 to 70% starch concentration.

For instance, millet flour that comes from millet seeds brings with it a 70% starch concentration. On the other hand, with sorghum flour, you get a 68% starch concentration. This is also the same with white flours that bring a 68% starch concentration to your meal.

No doubt, these various food items sometimes come with their benefits and nutrients. However, the reality is that the risk that it poses to you, thanks to its high starch concentration, far outweighs any benefit or nutrient it promises.

5. Oats – 57.9% Starch Concentration

The next food item on the list is oats. This is perhaps surprising considering that claims state that oats come with many benefits to the body. Unfortunately, you still need to contend with a high concentration of starch intake each time you consume oats.

Precisely, with every 81 grams of starch that you consume, you also consume 46.9 grams of starch.

6. Noodles – 56% Starch Concentration

This should not be a surprise addition to the list. However, just in case you did not know, noodles come with a high concentration of starch. Even more, they are quite low in starch and highly processed.

Each time you get a packet, you get 54 grams of carbohydrate. You also get 13.4 grams of fats. Now, out of the 54 grams of carbohydrate, you get 47.7 grams of it as starch. This is why it is extremely dangerous to the body, more so, its low nutrients make up.

For instance, reports show that individuals that consistently consume noodles are more likely to experience diabetes, heart diseases, and metabolic syndrome.

7. Bread & Bread Products – 40.2 to 44.4% Starch Concentration

As expected, bread and bread products are one food item that has a high concentration of starch. Examples of food items that fall under this category include bagels, white bread, tortillas, and English muffins.

In most cases, these products come from wheat flour, usually refined. They come with considerable starch that can spike the body's sugar level. For instance, English muffins come with 44.4% starch concentration. Bagels come with 43.6% starch concentration, while white bread comes with 40.8% starch concentration.

8. Shortbread Cookies – 40.5% Starch Concentration

This Scottish treat also possesses significant starch concentration. This is largely thanks to their constituents, sugar, flour, and butter. Typically, with a cookie of 12 grams, you get as much as 4.8 grams of starch from it. Even more, these commercial cookies sometimes contain artificial fats that increase the risk of diabetes, belly fat, and heart diseases.

9. Rice – 28.7% Starch Concentration

As you know, rice represents the most eaten staple food all around the globe. Unfortunately, it is far from healthy as it has a high concentration of starch. Typically, with rice, you get a 28.7% starch concentration.

Now, while this is already considerable, this amount increases significantly in cases of uncooked rice. With uncooked rice, you get as much as 63.6% starch in every gram consumed.

Worse, starch also has a high Glycemic index. In turn, it can comprise a human's mucous membrane. When this is compromised, it becomes only a matter of time before a wide range of health conditions begin to emerge in such individuals.

10. Pasta – 26% Starch Concentration

The next food item with a considerable starch concentration is pasta. This refers to a noodle type that comes from durum wheat. While it comes in various forms like macaroni, fettuccine, and spaghetti, the reality is that they all hold starch.

It comes with a high 26% starch concentration that makes it very unhealthy to your body system. Worse, this starch concentration increases to around 62.5% when it is uncooked.

11. Corn – 18.2% Starch Concentration

The next food item that contributes a significant starch amount to your body is corn. Unfortunately, it is also one of the most consumed cereal in the world. So, you can tell the number of damages it does to the human body.

Also, while corn stands as a vegetable, its starch constituents make it less desirable for consumption. With each cup of corn, you get 18.2% of it as starch. This is even more disturbing as, according to Dr. Sebi, what we now regard as corn is not a natural substance. Rather, it is one that has undergone genetic engineering.

12. Potatoes – 18% Starch Concentration

The final food item on this list is potato. This food is quite common in most homes, thanks to its versatility. Still, they have a significant amount of starch. No doubt, they do not hold as much starch as other food items on this list. However, they still come with an 18% concentration that is far from healthy, more so their high consumption in most homes.

Conclusion

Starch is one of the most consumed food substances today across the globe. In most cases, most people do not even acknowledge that they are engaging in high starch consumption. This is sometimes due to ignorance of food constituents and sometimes lack of concern for what goes into their body.

Unfortunately, the reality is that starch consumption is predominant, and it is far from ideal for the body. As Dr. Sebi has established, starch contains substances that are harmful to the body. It contains cyanide and arsenic acid that increases the acidity of the body. In turn, this acidic level interferes with the alkalinity balance of the body.

This imbalance is what makes the body a viable breeding ground for various diseases. As such, you must eliminate your starch intake or reduce it to the barest minimum if you intend to live a healthy life. In the next chapter, we will discuss mucus, its role in the body, and Dr. Sebi's view on it.

CHAPTER THREE

MUCUS

Introduction

The creation of mucus is an essential aspect of our bodies. Each day, the body constantly produces doses of mucus for a wide range of functions. Typically, this production is for the benefit of the body. Unfortunately, as with everything in life, it can become negative when the production becomes excessive.

This idea is one that underpins Dr. Sebi's road to a healthy diet. Unfortunately, there has been a misconstruction of the role of mucus within the body. Even worse, it continues to receive limited attention when it is, in fact, a core component of healthy living. Precisely, where the mucus membrane is allowed to function properly, it performs a wide range of functions that keep the body in the best condition possible.

On the other hand, where it is pressured due to a wide variety of activities, including poor diet, it results in excessive mucus production, making the body susceptible to illness. It is necessary that you understand the role of mucus in the body and the various dietary options that can compromise the mucus membrane.

What is mucus?

This refers to a stringy and slippery fluid substance that various lining tissues within the body produce. While this is sometimes perceived as unwanted, the reality is that mucus is actually essential to normal body functioning. This is because it performs a wide range of essential functions within critical organs.

Mucus has various components, with the most prominent being mucin. It is this mucin that works as a selective barrier, viscous material, or lubricant. In this case, the function it performs will depend on the mucin's structure.

Note that the body produces a significant amount of mucus. For instance, each day, it is estimated that the body produces a minimum of 1 liter. This can then rise to as much as 1.5 liters in some cases. However, the good news is that we hardly notice the production of this mucus. As we stated, they perform essential functions within the body that makes this significant production desirable.

The mucus gland is responsible for the production of mucus. It is located in various body sites and includes the lungs, sinuses, throat, nose, cervix, gastrointestinal tract, and mouth.

Mucus vs. Phlegm

It is important to differentiate between mucus and phlegm. This is thanks to the popular confusion among people. In numerous cases, most people tend to use both terms interchangeably. However, they are distinct.

As we discussed earlier, mucus is produced by the lining tissues within the body. Phlegm, on the other hand, is a type of mucus. It refers to mucus that the respiratory system produces when there is excess mucus production within the body. You usually cough it up as it clogs your airways and can lead to nasal congestion, among others.

As such, while phlegm is a type of mucus, it should not be confused with mucus generally. This is because phlegm is associated with excessive mucus production and necessarily unwanted in the body. Instead, mucus is a lining that provides protection and moisturizing effect within the body and is typically wanted.

The role of mucus in the body

Just as with every natural production within the body, mucus performs a wide range of functions within the body. Typically, these functions are positive and necessary for the proper functioning of the body system. The various roles that mucus performs in the body include:

It Acts as a Protective Layer

One of the primary roles of mucus is to act as a protective layer for various critical organs and body systems. As we mentioned above, mucus is a slippery substance that covers various organs within the body.

For instance, it stands in the lungs and covers the area, protecting it from bacteria, as you will find out below. It also protects it from irritants that can cause discomfort. This explains the significance of mucus as a protective layer within your body.

It Acts as a Moisturizing Layer

Another relevant function that mucus performs within the body is to act as a moisturizing layer. Naturally, various critical organs within the body need to remain moisturized to perform effectively. In some cases, they even need to be moisturized to remain functional. Well, mucus is one substance that discharges this function.

Thanks to its constituent, it ensures that these various organs do not dry out. It ensures that they remain hydrated, which allows these organs to continue functioning.

It Traps Irritants Within the Body

Each day, the body is faced with a wide range of irritants. These irritants can emerge in a wide range of body areas. Unfortunately, these irritants cause harm to the body. In fact, when our body is exposed to such irritants, it could cause a wide range of discomfort.

Eventually, this discomfort is what results in various conditions that you know today. For instance, irritants like smoke are what result in lung damage. This is because the smoke consistently irritates the area.

One substance that contributes to fighting off these irritants is mucus, and this is one of the functions of mucus within the body. It traps these various irritants such as bacteria, smoke, and dust. It then aids the body in expelling these irritants. This is the reason why many smokers, for example, have a frequent cough throughout the year. Their body is trying it's best to help get rid of this type of irritant.

Mucus contains various substances like protein, water, and salt. In turn, they can transport dead cells, debris, and dust away from the lungs and nose. They also transport unwanted substances out of the body through the stomach.

It fights off infections

Another prominent role that mucus performs within the body is to aid the fight against infections. This is thanks to its antibody composition and bacteria-killing enzymes. A combination of this ensures that the human body is less habitable for bacteria, which causes infection and disease.

Furthermore, thanks to the slippery nature of the mucus, it fights off bacteria by making attachment less possible. It makes it harder for bacteria to attach itself to various organs that result in infections.

Instead, as we discussed above, it traps these various bacteria, renders them immobile, such that there can be no aggregation. In turn, the absence of aggregation ensures that your body system enjoys better health as bacteria and other infections are less dangerous when they do not stick together.

Now, as you can see, mucus performs a wide range of positive functions within the body that allows you to retain good health.

The problem with mucus

So far, it has become more evident that mucus is not just a disgusting element that should not be in your body. Instead, it is a vital component that your body constantly produces to keep it in shape.

So, where does the problem come from, and how does this important body component become an issue? As we have illustrated so far, the body needs a constant balance of all its constituents to function effectively. Too little of an important component, and you will have a problem. On the other hand, too much of anything, and there is still a problem.

Think back to our discussion in chapter one, where we discussed the need to find a balance between alkaline and acidic intake. Well, this is also the case with mucus within the body.

While mucus performs a wide range of positive functions within the body, the problem arises when mucus production exceeds the natural level. As Dr. Sebi would rightly say, this causes a wide range of problems within the body. For instance, too much mucus within the joints becomes a problem. While the mucus should ordinarily hydrate the joint, it begins to cause issues, which we now know as arthritis.

Excessive mucus production becomes an issue as it brings discomfort in the various areas where it occurs. For instance, it can cause a runny nose, sore throat, cough, sinus headache, sore throat, and nasal congestion.

Western medicine would have you believe that excessive mucus rarely translates to a serious medical problem. However, as Dr. Sebi has established through his teachings, excessive mucus is, in fact, the cause of all diseases.

The presence of excessive mucus in the bronchial is what causes what we now know as bronchitis. If you are experiencing eye issues, then the brain is seeing more mucus production than it is healthy for it. So, it becomes evident that excessive production of mucus within the body is not just another issue. In fact, a serious issue deserves your attention.

What causes the excessive production of mucus?

Clearly, mucus is a substance that keeps the body performing and functioning effectively. On the other hand, it is also a substance that can result in significant health issues within the body where its production becomes excessive.

As such, it is necessary for you to ensure that the body production of mucus stays within the recommended limits. In turn, to ensure this, it is necessary to understand what causes excessive production of mucus. This is because when you understand what causes excessive production, you can take action to prevent it.

So, what are the factors that contribute to the excessive production of mucus? We will begin with the general causes of increased mucus production before diving into the core reason for such excessive production. This way, you can be fully equipped to maintain good health.

So, the various factors responsible for excessive mucus production include:

Respiratory infections

One of the most common reasons for mucus production within the body is respiratory infections. As always, our body is not always immune to infections. In turn, this infection can contribute to excessive mucus production, which makes us more vulnerable to other infections.

When it comes to respiratory infections, this involves various infections that affect the respiratory system. They include infections such as flu, cold, and sinusitis, among others. These various infections increase the rate of mucus production within the respiratory system. In turn, you will find yourself coughing up mucus when you have any of these infections.

You must have experienced it at least once a year, being unwell with a respiratory infection. You must have noticed that you had a thickened mucus that even appeared darker than usual. In some cases, the mucus was also yellow-green. Well, this is a result of increased mucus production within your body.

Allergic reactions

Another reason why mucus production will increase significantly is thanks to the existence or occurrence of allergic reactions within the body. Typically, allergic reactions push your body outside of its natural state. In turn, this can lead the body to react through the increased production of mucus.

Now, where this allergic reaction persists, it will only result in mucus's excessive production within the body. Note that when it comes to allergic reactions, cause of it hardly matters. As long as the body begins to function outside its natural state, increased mucus production occurs.

For instance, eating spicy foods when one is allergic to them would not negate this rule. While spicy foods are believed to ease up nasal congestion from mucus, this will not be the case if you are allergic to it. In such a case, the allergic food – spicy food – will only significantly increase mucus production.

Toxins and pollutants

Another factor responsible for the increased production of mucus in humans is toxins and pollutants. When it comes to toxins and pollutants, it involves a wide range of environmental factors that pollute the body system—for instance, living in an environment that sees an increased production of carbon monoxide and other pollutants like smoke will surely increase mucus production.

Similarly, living in a dry environment will usually spur the transmission of toxins in the air. This is thanks to the increased presence of dust within the environment. This becomes even more considerable where the environment is indoors. This, in turn, can leave the body in a polluted state, which will cause the mucus membrane to overcompensate when producing mucus.

In some other cases, this might be the willful intake of various toxins into the body. For instance, constant smoking is one event that sees the release of toxins into our bodies. These toxins, in turn, affect our respiratory system and lymphatic system. This then causes the increased production of mucus within those areas and the body at large.

This is very straightforward when you consider the case of smokers. In most cases, you find them having lung issues. This is because due to the intake of toxins, the mucus membrane is forced to overproduce mucus. In turn, this has its toll on the body system resulting in what we now tag as lung issues.

Dietary practices

The final and core factor that contributes to the excessive production of mucus is your dietary practice. This stands as the core factor because it gives rise to excessive mucus production in most cases. Furthermore, this is one area that you are directly responsible for, and you can effectively avoid.

As we have repeatedly stated, your diet plays a huge role in whether you maintain a healthy living or otherwise. Well, this extends to the production of mucus within the body. What you eat each day will determine if you wake with excessive mucus production. Similarly, it will determine if you wake up with normal mucus production and feel good about yourself.

Typically, when it comes to dietary practices, what is responsible for the increased production of mucus is food additives. You must keep in mind that this is, unfortunately, the mainstay of most food options today. We constantly take preserved foods, among other acidic foods. This group of foods affects the respiratory system, gastrointestinal tract, and lymphatic system. In turn, this culminates in increased mucus production.

Top 12 mucus causing foods to avoid

As we have established above, a major reason for excessive mucus production is your dietary practices. Various food substances and beverages can cause your body to start producing mucus at an alarming rate. As you already know, this is hardly the best thing for your body.

However, it is also important to understand and identify those food substances that can result in mucus's excessive production within the body. This way, you can take necessary action to avoid them and keep the body in top condition. The top 12 foods you want to avoid are as follows:

1. Dairy Products

The first category of food that you want to avoid is dairy products. This involves various food options like milk and eggs. These products tend to increase the production of mucus in your body.

You can easily confirm this by assessing your phlegm. You will find out that in most cases, it results in thicker phlegm. Well, this is because there has been a significant increase in mucus production.

2. Soybeans Products

The next category of food to avoid is soybeans and other food products from it. Examples of such food products include tofu and soymilk. This is because these products come off as cold damp. In turn, they tend to increase mucus production within the body, just like dairy products.

3. Corn Products

Earlier in chapter two, we recommend that you avoid corn and its products thanks to its high concentration of starch. If you were not convinced to avoid corn products, then this is another reason to do so.

Corn products are not just high in starch. They also aid and contribute to the excessive production of mucus within the body. As such, you want to avoid the intake of corn into the body. This is even more important in cases where you are already suffering from respiratory infections that ordinarily increases mucus production.

Now, eating any of these prohibited products will not only see a spike in the production of mucus. Thanks to the already existing spike, it will result in a wide range of

health issues across your body, disturbing your good
health.

4. Sugary Treats

One food that we enjoy is sugary treats. They take
different forms but are characterized by the considerable
presence of sugar in them. They may also come in the
form of food products with a significant presence of
refined sugars in them. Popular examples of these sugary
treats include cakes, cookies, pies, pastries, and sweets.

These substances are bad for your health as they
contribute significantly to mucus's excessive production
within the body. So, you want to ensure that you stay clear
of them, especially in a time like this.

5. Oily Foods

It would be best to also avoid oily foods. These food
substances are fried with oil. This also tends to contribute
to the significant production of mucus in the body. This
will include food substances like buns, bagels, muffins,
and pretzels.

You might be wondering why this food is a problem.
Well, this is thanks to the fact that it contains a significant
amount of oil. The body finds it difficult to digest these
food substances. When the body does, what occurs is that
the gastrointestinal tract witnesses a significant increase in
mucus, which puts your body at risk.

6. Oils

You might be wondering what the difference between this and the category identified above is. This category differs because it involves oils themselves. In the case of the above, it involves general food substances that you cook in oil. However, in this case, it concerns oils such as sunflower, safflower, and even sesame oil.

With this option, you consume a food substance that has a considerable presence of omega-six fatty acids. Now, these are unsaturated fats that can significantly increase the rate at which your body produces mucus. So, you want to avoid this food option.

7. Jams and Peanut Butter

The fact is that jams and peanut butter are the last things your body wants as a meal. They contain various sugar components that can weaken the presence of good bacteria within the body. In turn, this will only leave your body more vulnerable and increase the production of mucus within your body.

No doubt, they are a tasty category of food. However, your body's health remains the priority and if that is the case, then avoid them.

8. Nuts

Another food substance that does no good to our body system is nuts. They are known to increase the production of mucus within the body significantly. In turn, you will find yourself suffering from a sore throat. It can even become quite worse if you are one who is allergic to nuts.

You do not want to take any risk with your health. So, avoid this mucus causing food.

9. Salty and Fatty Foods

Over the course of this list, we have mentioned the need to avoid food cooked with oils. We also mentioned the need to avoid these unnatural oils themselves. Well, that is not all.

Another food substance that can cause excessive production of mucus within your body is salty and fatty foods. Various studies have shown that individuals that consume fatty and salty foods witness more occurrences of phlegm.

Well, this is thanks to the increased production of mucus within the body. In turn, the constant consumption of salty and fatty foods will only do more damage than good. So, to avoid excessive accumulation of mucus within the body, it is necessary to avoid salty and fatty foods.

10. Alcohol

There is a wide variety of reasons why it is ill advised to consume alcohol. While you might think that something like alcohol has nothing to do with the excessive production of mucus within the body, that is far from the case.

In fact, we can attribute mucus overproduction within the body to alcohol. This is because the intake of alcohol causes dehydration within the body. In turn, the moisturizing capacity of the mucus is significantly reduced. In turn, to compensate, there is an increased mucus production, which results in more harm than good.

For instance, you find that those that consume alcohol have a significant amount of thick phlegm in their lungs. They will even have problems coughing it up, which leads to a wide range of lung issues.

As such, to keep the body in good condition and maintain the balance of mucus production, it is necessary to avoid alcohol.

11. Caffeine

Caffeine is quite popular today among most households. Even as an individual, you will sometimes find yourself taking as much as one to three cups of caffeine in one day. Unfortunately, this is one food intake that contributes significantly to the overproduction of mucus within the body.

This becomes even more severe when you regularly consume your caffeine with milk or tea. As we mentioned earlier, dairy products also contribute to the overproduction of mucus in the body. So, combining them is sure to make things worse for everybody.

12. Carbonated Drinks and Beverages

Finally, you also want to avoid carbonated drinks and beverages. These food substances are full of preservatives and additives that affect the respiratory system and the gastrointestinal tract. So, you want to avoid this food substance at all costs.

Note that this list is not exhaustive of the various food substances that cause mucus's overproduction within the body. Other food substances contribute to it. For instance, we have wheat products and other processed foods.

Conclusion

The importance of diet for your body cannot be overstated. It plays a significant role in whether your body enjoys the best health or otherwise. As such, it is necessary to pay attention to it.

While mucus in the body is inevitable, more so, its importance, maintaining a balanced production is even more important. This is because the overproduction of mucus is associated with a wide range of health issues.

It is your responsibility to ensure that you avoid foods that contribute to mucus overproduction. In the next chapter, we will provide an overview of the alkaline diet and the importance of getting the right pH balance.

CHAPTER FOUR

WHAT IS THE ALKALINE DIET? WHY IS PH BALANCE IMPORTANT?

Introduction

The body is in constant need of balance. Each day, the various body systems work to keep this balance in place through the release, processing, and cleansing of substances from the body system.

If this balance is lost, the body begins to degenerate. In the long run, there is overproduction and accumulation of mucus within the body and becomes only a matter of time before the body begins to manifest with a wide range of diseases and issues.

From the preceding, it becomes evident that good health becomes more than guaranteed once you secure the balance within the body. However, while this is clear and you understand the need to maintain balance within the body, one thing remains unclear; this is how to maintain this balance.

In recent times, a wide range of medications and activities have emerged as a means to achieve this. In some cases, unsuccessful. In others, partly unsuccessful. Regardless, the need for the body's balance remains as pressing as ever.

One way of being sure to achieve this successfully is through Dr. Sebi's alkaline diet. Note that this was the underlying advice in Dr. Sebi's teachings on dietary practices. According to him, all that the body needs to retain its health status is an alkaline diet. While this seemed far-fetched at first, it becomes apparent that this is the case.

What is an alkaline diet?

The idea behind an alkaline diet is the consumption of alkaline foods. As we discussed in chapter one, the body constantly needs to balance its acidic level and alkalinity level. Even more, the balance must be one in favor of alkalinity, as the body needs to have as much as 80% alkalinity level compared to the 20% acidic level.

In a nutshell, an alkaline diet involves consuming foods that ensure there is adequate alkalinity within the body (by consuming alkaline foods, such as leafy greens, avocados and quinoa) and reduced acidity (by avoiding packet and processed foods, read meats, coffee and alcohol). This will ensure that the body can combat a wide range of diseases and retain the best health possible.

This dietary practice is also known as the alkaline diet or acid-alkaline diet. It stipulates that what you take in daily goes a long way in determining your body's pH level. It recommends the consumption of alkaline foods to ensure that the pH level within the body stays alkaline rather than acidic.

Understanding the Ph level of the body

Now, it is vital that you understand what the pH level with the body means. It involves the measurement of the body's alkalinity and acidity. The lower the pH level, the higher the acidity of the body. On the other hand, the higher the number on the scale, the more alkaline your body is.

The pH level of the body is measured on a scale of 0 to 14. At one end is the acidic level. On the other end is the alkaline level. Now, in the middle is the neutral state where the body is neither acidic nor alkaline. Here is the range:

- Acidic: Ranges from 0.0 to 6.9

- Neutral: Stands at 7.0

- Alkaline: Ranges from 7.1 to 14.0

Furthermore, you must understand that the body does not hold just one pH level. Precisely, the pH level across various body systems differs. For instance, some parts are naturally acidic, while some other parts are alkaline.

Take, for example, your stomach. It is naturally acidic. In fact, it stands between the pH level of 2 to 3.5. This is thanks to the presence of hydrochloric acid within the body. However, this acid is indispensable within the body as it is necessary for the digestion of food.

So, the stomach cannot be alkaline. In such a case, there will be no digestion within the body system, which will only result in death.

On the other hand, the blood is naturally alkaline, although slightly. It has a pH level between 7.36 and 7.44. This allows it to function effectively. In fact, your blood's failure to maintain this pH level is fatal as it would result in severe health conditions in most cases and mostly death.

So, it becomes necessary for the body's pH balance to retain its natural state for the proper functioning of all body systems.

Understanding the Ph in food

No doubt, you have established that the pH balance of the body is important. While we would discuss the reason for this importance in detail, you must understand the pH in foods.

As earlier discussed in chapter one, the food you consume plays a significant role in your body's pH level. That is why it is essential that you understand the pH in food. However, note that this is different from pH and food.

When it comes to pH and food, we focus on the capacity of food substances to affect the body's pH level. However, when it comes to pH in food, it concerns the pH level of food itself.

Although we have earlier listed out acidic and alkaline food substances in the chapter, it is largely insufficient unless you gain a full understanding of the relationship between food and its pH level. Now, what are we talking about?

Every food substance comes with its pH level. The scale above is also applicable in determining whether a food substance is acidic or alkaline. However, that is only half of the equation.

What determines whether a food substance is acidic or alkaline is not only its pH level when tested outside the body. Instead, it involves its reaction when within the body. Note that this is very important in understanding whether a food is acidic or alkaline.

This is because while food might be tested as acidic in the natural environment, it might function otherwise when in the body. This usually occurs during the digestion stages of such food.

For example, lemons are naturally acidic in nature. They contain citric acid, which has a pH of around 2.0 to 3.0. However, upon consumption, they turn out to be among the most alkalizing food out there. This is also the case with Brussel sprouts and kimchi.

So, it is vital that you keep in mind that the original pH of a food is not always final in determining whether it is acidic or alkaline. You must also consider the likelihood of changes in the food's pH upon introduction into the body.

Other examples of food substances changing their pH level after getting into the body include:

- **Fresh lemon:** from between 2.0 and 3.0 to 10.0 after getting into the body

- **Brussel sprouts:** from 6.3 to 10.0 after getting into the body

- **Kimchi**: from 4.2 to 10.0 after getting into the body

- **Raw spinach**: from 6.8 to 10.0 after getting into the body

- **Watermelon**: from between 5.2 and 5.8 to 9.5 after getting into the body

- **Broccoli**: from 6.5 to 9.5 after getting into the body

- **Kale**: from between 6.4 and 6.8 to 9.5 after getting into the body

- **Celery:** from between 5.7 and 6.0 to 9.0 after getting into the body

- **Blackberries**: from between 3.8 and 4.5 to 8.5 after getting into the body

- **Apricots**: from between 3.3 and 4.8 to 8.5 after getting into the body

- **Onions**: from between 5.3 and 5.8 to 8.5 after getting into the body

- **Ginseng**: from between 6.0 and 6.5 to 8.5 after getting into the body

- **Ginger**: from between 5.6 and 5.9 to 8.5 after getting into the body

- **Garlic**: from 5.8 to 8.5 after getting into the body

- **Carrots**: from between 5.8 and 6.4 to 8.5 after getting into the body

- **Alfalfa**: from 6.0 to 8.5 after getting into the body

- **Passion fruit:** from between 3.0 and 3.2 to 8.5 after getting into the body

- **Papaya**: from between 5.2 and 6.0 to 8.5 after getting into the body

- **Pears**: from between 3.5 and 4.6 to 8.5 after getting into the body

- **Nectarines**: from between 3.9 and 4.1 to 8.5 after getting into the body

- **Kiwis fruit**: from between 3.1 and 3.9 to 8.5 after getting into the body

- **Grapes**: from between 2.9 and 3.8 to 8.5 after getting into the body

- **Grapefruit**: from between 3.0 and 3.7 to 8.5 after getting into the body

- **Figs**: from between 5.0 and 5.9 to 8.5 after getting into the body

- **Dates**: from between 4.1 and 4.8 to 8.5 after getting into the body

- **Chestnuts**: from 5.9 to 7.5 after getting into the body

- **Chives**: from between 5.2 and 6.3 to 7.5 after getting into the body

- **Bamboo shoots**: from between 5.1 and 6.2 to 7.5 after getting into the body

- **Strawberries**: from between 3.0 and 3.9 to 7.5 after getting into the body

- **Guava**: from 5.5 to 7.5 after getting into the body

- **Blueberries**: from between 3.1 and 3.3 to 7.5 after getting into the body

- **Almonds**: from 6.9 to 8.0 after getting into the body

- **Wild rice**: from between 6.0 and 6.4 to 8.0 after getting into the body

- **Turnips**: from between 5.2 and 5.5 to 8.0 after getting into the body

- **Tomato**: from between 4.2 and 4.9 to 8.0 after getting into the body

- **Olives**: from between 6.0 and 7.0 to 8.0 after getting into the body

- **Pumpkin**: from between 4.9 and 5.5 to 8.0 after getting into the body

- **Mushrooms**: from between 6.0 and 6.7 to 8.0 after getting into the body

- **Green cabbage**: from between 5.5 and 6.7 to 8.0 after getting into the body

- **Cauliflower**: from 5.6 and 8.0 after getting into the body

- **Peppers**: from between 4.5 and 5.4 to 8.0 after getting into the body

- **Peaches**: from between 3.3 and 4.0 to 8.0 after getting into the body

- **Oranges**: from between 3.6 and 4.3 to 8.0 after getting into the body

- **Apples**: from between 3.3 and 4.0 to 8.0 after getting into the body

The At-A-Glance Acid/Alkaline Food List

EAT MORE   EAT LESS

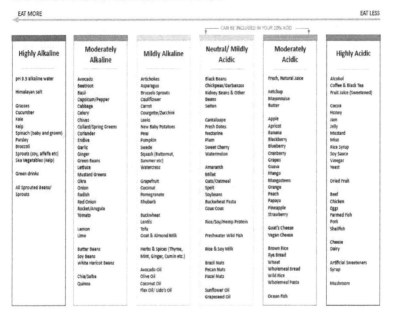

—— CAN BE INCLUDED IN YOUR 20% ACID ——

Highly Alkaline	Moderately Alkaline	Mildly Alkaline	Neutral/ Mildly Acidic	Moderately Acidic	Highly Acidic
pH 9.5 alkaline water	Avocado	Artichokes	Black Beans	Fresh, Natural Juice	Alcohol
	Beetroot	Asparagus	Chickpeas/Garbanzos		Coffee & Black Tea
Himalayan salt	Basil	Brussels Sprouts	Kidney Beans & Other	Ketchup	Fruit Juice (Sweetened)
	Capsicum/Pepper	Cauliflower	Beans	Mayonnaise	
Grasses	Cabbage	Carrot	Seitan	Butter	Cocoa
Cucumber	Celery	Courgette/Zucchini			Honey
Kale	Chives	Leeks	Cantaloupe	Apple	Jam
Kelp	Collard/Spring Greens	New Baby Potatoes	Fresh Dates	Apricot	Jelly
Spinach (baby and grown)	Coriander	Peas	Nectarine	Banana	Mustard
Parsley	Endive	Pumpkin	Plum	Blackberry	Miso
Broccoli	Garlic	Swede	Sweet Cherry	Blueberry	Rice Syrup
Sprouts (soy, alfalfa etc)	Ginger	Squash (Butternut,	Watermelon	Cranberry	Soy Sauce
Sea Vegetables (Kelp)	Green Beans	Summer etc)		Grapes	Vinegar
	Lettuce	Watercress	Amaranth	Guava	Yeast
Green drinks	Mustard Greens		Millet	Mango	
	Okra	Grapefruit	Oats/Oatmeal	Mangosteen	Dried Fruit
All Sprouted Beans/	Onion	Coconut	Spelt	Orange	
Sprouts	Radish	Pomegranate	Soybeans	Peach	Beef
	Red Onion	Rhubarb	Buckwheat Pasta	Papaya	Chicken
	Rocket/Arugula		Cous Cous	Pineapple	Eggs
	Tomato	Buckwheat		Strawberry	Farmed Fish
		Lentils	Rice/Soy/Hemp Protein		Pork
	Lemon	Tofu		Goat's Cheese	Shellfish
	Lime	Goat & Almond Milk	Freshwater Wild Fish	Vegan Cheese	
					Cheese
	Butter Beans	Herbs & Spices (Thyme,	Rice & Soy Milk	Brown Rice	Dairy
	Soy Beans	Mint, Ginger, Cumin etc.)		Rye Bread	
	White Haricot Beans		Brazil Nuts	Wheat	Artificial Sweeteners
		Avocado Oil	Pecan Nuts	Wholemeal Bread	Syrup
	Chia/Salba	Olive Oil	Hazel Nuts	Wild Rice	
	Quinoa	Coconut Oil		Wholemeal Pasta	Mushroom
		Flax Oil/ Udo's Oil	Sunflower Oil		
			Grapeseed Oil	Ocean Fish	

Why is Ph balance important?

The importance of the pH balance within the body cannot be overestimated. If you have been following through with us, you would have realized that this balance goes a long way in determining whether a person is healthy or otherwise.

Let us illustrate the underlying notion that makes the pH balance so important.

Now, the breakdown of food within your body involves the conversion or transformation of food substances within the body into energy. This process is quite similar to a fire. This is because there is a chemical reaction responsible for the breakdown of solid mass in both cases.

However, unlike fire, the chemical reaction within the body occurs in a controlled manner and slowly. So, the breakdown of food involves a step-by-step process.

Now, once you eat food, and it gets broken down, it always leaves a residue. This residue is called metabolic waste. You can better understand it by remembering that once a fire completes the burning process, it leaves ash residue behind. In the case of food breakdown, the ash residue left behind is what we referred to as metabolic waste earlier.

This metabolic waste takes the nature of the food substance that you consume. As such, it can either be acidic, neutral, or alkaline. Consequently, the metabolic waste within your body reflects the food you consume and the pH balance of your body.

If you have an already acidic pH level and you take acidic foods, your metabolic waste will be acidic. However, it does not stop there. This metabolic waste goes on to significantly affect the pH level of your body. Such that, the acidic metabolic waste makes your body even more acidic.

As discussed in chapter one, an acidic body comes with significant health issues, including unhealthy skin, hair and nails, digestive issues, mouth and teeth issues, complications with the nervous system, and eyes, head, and general body discomfort.

On the other hand, where you consume alkaline foods in an alkaline body system, the advantage is numerous. This is because the body's metabolic waste goes on to be alkaline in nature. In turn, it allows the blood to retain the necessary alkaline level, which keeps the body in top condition.

So, from the illustration, it becomes evident that the body's pH balance is important because it affects the subsequent alkalinity of the blood. Then, it determines whether the body retains its ability to function effectively.

Beyond this, other reasons why the body's pH balance is important includes:

- It allows you to maintain a healthy body weight and experience weight loss where necessary

- It allows you to improve your body's ability to absorb mineral and vitamins

- It allows you to reduce the magnesium deficiencies within the body

- It allows you to improve the functioning of your immune system

- It allows you to reduce the potential of experiencing cancer

- It allows you to reduce the risk of various heart problems and diseases, including stroke

- It allows you to improvise your muscle mass and bone density

- It allows you to improve the various functioning of your organs

- It allows you to support a healthier blood Keep in mind that this list is in no way exhaustive of the various reasons why keeping your body's pH balance is vital. However, you need to take from here that keeping the pH level in a balanced state is very integral to a safe and healthy life.

Conclusion

Western medicine would have you believe that the food you take does not affect the pH level of your blood. According to western medicine, all it affects is your urine. Your blood and body system has a way of regulating itself.

However, this is far from the case. If this were truly the case, then there would be no issues of heart problems and cancer that has now become an epidemic. You should know that your dietary practices significantly affect the pH balance of your body.

It is your responsibility to ensure that you maintain the best dietary practice that keeps your pH balance. This is not only integral for your short-term health. Instead, it is also integral for your long-term health. As such, take responsibility and prioritize alkalizing foods. This way, you can enjoy the good health that you desire.

In the next chapter, we will look at the top 10 alkaline foods.

CHAPTER FIVE

DR. SEBI'S TOP ALKALINE FOODS

Introduction

One thing that has been constant so far is the importance of alkaline foods to maintain the best health. This involves various food substances that provide an alkalizing effect within the body.

While we have identified the relevance and importance of these food substances, it is not enough. It is more important to understand and identify these various foods substances to ensure that you can effectively transition from a western diet to an alkaline-based diet.

So, here are the various top foods recommended by Dr. Sebi. We have divided these food substances into multiple categories. This ensures that you can quickly identify the appropriate food substances that you need to prioritize moving forward.

Vegetables

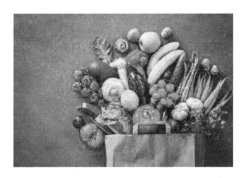

Examples of food options under this category include:

- Amaranth greens, also known as Callaloo

- Nopales, also known as Mexican cactus

- Mushrooms apart from Shitake

- Lettuce apart from Iceberg

- Kale

- Izote, also known as the cactus leaf or cactus flower

- Garbanzo beans

- Dandelion greens

- Cucumber

- Chayote, also known as Mexican squash

- Bell peepers

- Avocado

- Wild arugula

- Purslane (verdolaga)

- Watercress

- Turnip greens

- Zucchini

- Tomatillo

- Squash

- Tomato although only plum and cherry options

- Onions

- Sea vegetables

  (dulse/arame/inori/hijiki/wakame)

- Okra

- Olives

Fruits

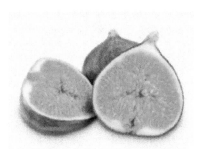

Examples of food options under this category include:

- Mango

- Limes (ensure they are key limes with seeds)

- Seeded grapes

- Figs

- Dates

- Currants

- Cherries

- Cantaloupe

- Any form of elder elderberries

- All varieties of berries except cranberries

- The smallest bananas, original banana, midsize banana, and Burro

- Peaches

- Tamarind

- Soursops from the West Indian or Latin markets

- Soft jelly coconuts

- Seeded raisins

- Prunes

- Prickly bear also known as cactus fruit

- Plums

- Pears

- Seeded melons

- Sour or Seville orange

Natural herbal teas

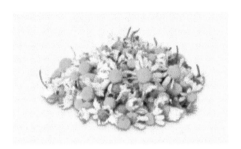

Examples of food options under this category include:

- Tila

- Raspberry

- Ginger

- Fennel

- Elderberry

- Chamomile

- Burdock

Grains

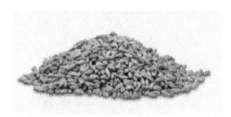

Examples of food options under this category include:

- Wild rice

- Tef

- Spelt

- Rye

- Quinoa

- Kamut

- Fonio Amaranth

Nuts and seeds

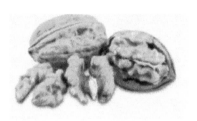

Examples of food options under this category include:

- Brazil Nuts

- Walnuts

- Raw sesame butter

- Raw sesame seeds

- Hemp seeds

Oils

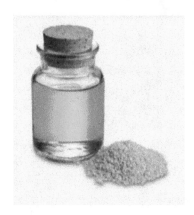

Examples of food options under this category include:

- Avocado oil

- Hemp seed oil

- Sesame oil

- Grapeseed oil

- Coconut oil (however, ensure that you do not cook it)

- Olive oil (however, ensure that you do not cook it)

Spices and seasonings

We can classify this category into four subcategories. They include:

Mild Favors

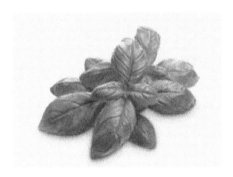

Examples of food options under this category include:

- Thyme
- Tarragon
- Sweet basil
- Savory
- Oregano
- Dill
- Cloves
- Bay leaf
- Basil

Salty Flavors

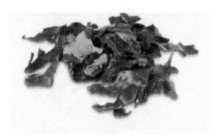

Examples of food options under this category include:

- Powdered, granulated seaweed

- Pure sea salt

- Nori/Dulse/Kelp

Sweet Flavors

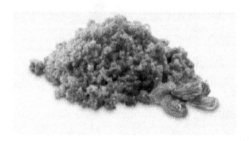

Examples of food options under this category include:

- Date sugar

- Pure agave syrup

Pungent and Spicy Flavors

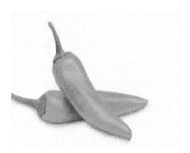

Examples of food options under this category include:

- Sage

- Habanero

- Onion powder

- Cayenne, also known as African Bird Pepper

- Achiote

Conclusion

Various food options allow you to keep within the alkaline diet. Th e good news is that these food options are viable. In turn, it ensures that you have a wide range of options to choose from and maintain a healthy body.

In the next chapter, we will discuss how to various alkaline diet recipes that will allow you to eliminate toxins from your body.

CHAPTER SIX

ALKALINE DIET RECIPES THAT WILL ELIMINATE TOXINS AND DISEASES FROM YOUR BODY

Introduction

Getting into an alkaline diet can seem like a severe restriction. This is due to the limited number of food substances that you are allowed to eat. There is no doubt that these restrictions are necessary for your body to remain in the best possible condition.

However, that is not our only concern. Our concerns also extend to ensuring that you can easily abide by diet rules under the alkaline-based diet. One way to achieve this is to ensure that the various food options can get transformed into a tasty meal.

Earlier, well listed various food options across different categories that you can consume. However, as you are new to the alkaline based diet, you are left to wonder how that becomes a meal that you can consume. We will introduce you to values recipes that you can maximize to create a meal from the various food options we discussed in the previous chapter.

Alkaline Diet Recipes

Various recipe options allow you to transform the previous chapter's food substances into a full-fledged meal. For better use and understanding, we will divide these various recipes into different categories based on the type of food they can function.

However, keep in mind that a recipe coming under a particular category does not mean that is the only category it applies to. In some instances, it can apply to more than one category. For instance, a recipe that falls under breakfast may also function as lunch.

Breakfast

1. Walnut Pear Salad

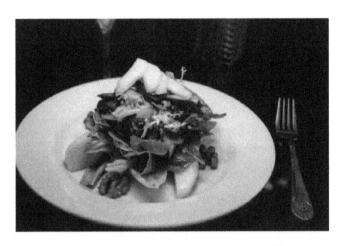

FALL PEAR WALNUT SALAD

Th is salad combines walnuts, juicy pears, and wild arugula to provide a great meal. With a touch of classy dressing, you are in line to enjoy a wonderful meal. **Ingredients**

- Walnut halves: ½ cup

- Agave syrup: ¼ cup

- Wild arugula: 8 large handfuls

- Pears: 2

- Olive oil: 4 tablespoons

- Key lime juice: ¼ cup

- Sea salt: a small pinch

Cooking Instructions

- Preheat your oven to around 350 degrees Fahrenheit

- Add the pinch of sea salt to the walnuts and mix with one tablespoon of the agave syrup

- Spread it within the oven and bake between 7 and 8 minutes. Once it is golden, remove it from the oven, then allow it to cool

- Now, add the remaining agave syrup along with the key lime juice, olive oil, and pinch of sea salt. Place it all into a jar and shake well after covering it

- Wash your pear and cut them lengthways into two. Now, remove their cores using a teaspoon and create long thin slices from each half

- Place the sliced pear and arugula into a large bowl of salad. Then, sprinkle the walnuts that must have cooled down. You can then add the dressing, and you are ready to eat

Lunch

1. Plant-Based Tacos

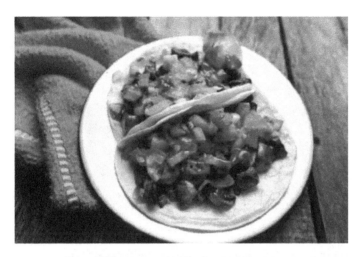

DR. SEBI'S PORTOBELLO TACOS

This is a smoky and spicy plant-based taco that brings taste and flavor all in one spoon **Ingredients**

- Portobello mushroom: 2 large
- Bell peppers: 2
- Red onion: ½
- Chopped cherry tomatoes: 1 cup
- Kamut flour tortillas: 8
- Key lime: 1

- Cayenne pepper and sea salt

- Grapeseed oil: ½ cup

- Avocado

Cooking Instructions

- Preheat your oven to around 425 degrees Fahrenheit

- Cut your portobello into half thick wedges

- Cut your onions into half-moons or half thick rings

- Slice the bell pepper into half thick strips

- Brush the mushrooms' sides, onions, tomatoes, and bell pepper with grapeseed oil. However, ensure the bulk of it goes to the mushroom

- Sprinkle your portobello with cayenne pepper or sea salt

- Roast until the portobello becomes tender. This should take around 20 minutes

- Warm your tortillas when it is time to use rice and divide the vegetables and portobello

- Serve the meal with key lime and avocado

Dinner

1. Alkaline Italian Pasta

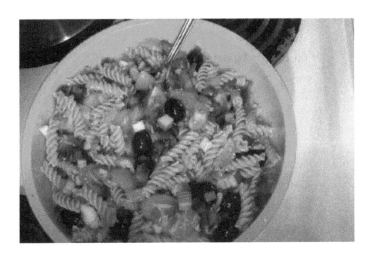

Th is Alkaline Italian Pasta allows you to combine the flavor of the black olives, Italian dressing, and an approved pasta to produce a spicy taste

Ingredients

- Springwater

- Dr. Sebi's approved pasta

- Cherry tomatoes

- Green pepper

- Red onion

- Bell pepper

- Black olives (do not buy then in a can)
- Italian dressing: ¼ cup

Cooking Instructions

- Start boiling your spring water and allows it to get heated up. Then, you can add your approved pasta

- Chop your cherry tomatoes into four. You can use as many as you want based on your pasta amount

- Chop your green pepper, red onion, and bell pepper into smaller pieces

- Once your pasta is ready, you can drain the water out and allow it to cool down

- Now add all the pepper, cherry tomato, onion, and olives into the pasta, which should be in a bowl now

- Shake the Italian dressing and add it to the bowl

- Now stir it carefully to ensure that your tomatoes remain in good shape

- Allow the Italian dressing to simmer, and your Alkaline Italian Pasta is ready

Dessert

1. Roasted Quinoa

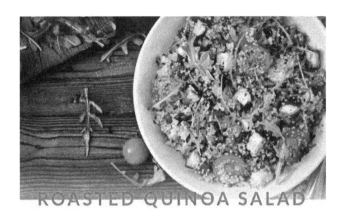

This roasted quinoa brings the taste and delicacy of the quinoa and combines it with the wild arugula with spectacular effect

Ingredients:

- Vegetable broth: 2 ½ cups

- Sea salt: 2 teaspoons

- Quinoa: 2 cups

- Green bell pepper: 2

- Diced and cored red bell pepper

- Chunks of zucchini

- Grapeseed oil: 2 tablespoons

- Seal salt

- Wild arugula: 3 cups

- Avocado: 1

- Red onion

Cooking Instructions

- Preheat your oven to around 400 degrees Fahrenheit

- Combine the salt and broth add to allow it to simmer while using medium heat

- Stir the quinoa and allow it to simmer. You can reduce the heat and allow it all to simmer for around 2o minutes

- Remove it from the fire and allow it cool until you are ready to serve it

- Now, fluff your quinoa properly just before serving

- As the quinoa simmer, add the zucchini and bell pepper to a pan and include olive sea salt and olive oil

- Roast for between 10 and 12 minutes until it is tender, and you can see that golden look

- Fold the quinoa but toss in the avocado and onion before this, and your meal is ready

Snacks

1. Nut and Banana Muffins

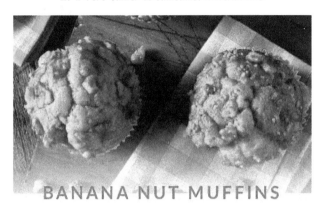

BANANA NUT MUFFINS

This recipe combines the benefits of bananas and nuts to provide a great snack for you

Ingredients

- Approved flour: 1 ½ cups

- Date sugar: ¾ cups

- Sea salt: ½ teaspoon

- Medium ripe mashed burro bananas: 2

- Walnut milk (homemade): ¾ cup

- Grapeseed oil: ¼ cup

- Key lime juice: 1 tablespoon

- Medium ripe chunks burro bananas: 1

- Chopped walnuts with extra sprinkles: ½ cup

Cooking Instructions

- Preheat your oven to around 400 degrees Fahrenheit

- Grease the muffin pan cups lightly

- Mix all dry ingredients in a bowl

- Mix the wet ingredients with the mashed bananas in another bowl

- Add the wet mixture to the dry mixture and mix them till they come alive. However, ensure that you do not over mix it

- Add the walnuts and chopped bananas and stir for three more times

- Divide it evenly across your muffin pan. You can always sprinkle extra walnuts

- Bake the nut and Banana muffins between 22 and 26 minutes

- Once you can see the golden-brown color around the edges, put a toothpick into the muffin. If it comes out clean, then it is ready

- Remove it and wait for around 10 minutes to allows it cool, then you can serve

Conclusion

You can combine the food options using various recipes to provide yourself a tasty meal. In turn, you can be sure to enjoy a better experience with an alkaline plant-based diet.

CHAPTER SEVEN

STARTING THE HEALING PROCESS: FROM WESTERN DIET TO ALKALINE BASED FOODS

Introduction

Just like the majority of us out there, you have mostly spent your life eating based on a western modern diet. That is a lot of potatoes in your meal, carbonated drinks and soda, and preservatives.

This has surely contributed to making your body a haven for infections and a wide range of other diseases. The good news is that you have realized it. In turn, you can transition from that unhealthy diet to a healthy one that keeps your body in the best possible condition. You can now move from the western-based diet to the alkaline plant-based diet.

With this, you can begin to rid your body of all the acidic metabolic waste that disrupts your body's pH balance. Even more, you can rid your body of excess mucus and maintain only the required mucus production that keeps your body in good health.

Starting the healing process

Over the years, the western diet has become more popular than ever. It easily fits into a lifestyle where people are less concerned about what they eat than they are about eating. The goal is now to eat rather than eat the right and most healthy meal. In turn, this has seen a significant rise in the focus on dairy products, processed foods, and genetically modified foods.

However, if you have followed through with us, one thing is clear about the consumption of these types of foods. They are far from the first thing our body is comfortable with. Still, we keep feeding our bodies with these substances. This then allows our body to become less healthy. You will find that there has been a significant increase in various health issues around the world following the increasing adherence to the western diet.

As we have now highlighted the dangers associated with the western diet, it is not enough to recognize these dangers; you must also take steps to prevent them. Even more, you must take steps to heal your body following previous years of bad eating habits that have damaged it.

Starting your healing process involves getting rid of various toxic food substances that you consume. You will also need to do away with various acidic food substances that have become the mainstay of the western diet and your existing diet. As we have established, these food substances cause the buildup of mucus. Even more, they result in chronic inflammation amidst a wide range of other chronic diseases.

Scientific evidence has established that these food substances are harmful to the human body. For instance, according to the World Health Organization, processed meat is carcinogenic to the human body. Even more, red meat is no exception as it is also classified as probably carcinogenic. There have also been other studies that establish that animal fat and animal protein increases the risk of heart diseases, diabetes, cancer, among other chronic conditions and illnesses.

You must transition to a plant-based diet to begin the homeostasis and healing of the body and its organs. This is the foundation and basis of good health. We must revert to natural and non-hybrid plant foods and herbs that support our natural body systems.

Typically, these plant foods are indigenous to Africa and other regions that share similar conditions with Africa. For instance, India, the Caribbean, South, and Central America. This is because these food substances grow under similar conditions that supported the development of the African genome, the foundation of the human genome.

According to Dr. Sebi, by maintaining only the consumption of these natural food substances, we can begin to rid our body of acidity. In turn, we can restore and maintain the required alkalinity level to guarantee our good health and wellbeing.

Now, as you begin your healing process, here is a list of food based on Dr. Sebi's recommendation that should help you rid your body of acidity.

Water

While we sometimes underestimate water's function within the body, the reality is that it plays a significant role. It contributes a huge deal to ensure that the human genome enjoys a natural expression that keeps it in good shape. As such, you must maintain a healthy consumption of water.

Keep in mind that fruits and vegetables are a great medium to provide the body with adequate water. This is because they contain a high concentration of fluids. Unfortunately, the consumption of fruits and vegetables is not prioritized under the western diet.

To begin your healing process, you must begin to take adequate water. In fact, you need as much as one gallon of water each day. This cut across both drinking water and the water in food. So, ensure you drink adequate water each day.

You do not need to worry about the degree of consumption as long as you exceed the one-gallon requirement. Your body can handle discharging the excess water through urine and other means.

It would be best to opt for spring water. This is because it contains a significant amount of natural minerals. In turn, this not only makes the water safe, but it also ensures that you can enjoy protection from harmful bacterial.

Also, avoid drinking tap water. This is because it contains chemicals such as chlorine designed to kill bacteria. It also contains fluoride that seeks to protect your teeth. Unfortunately, the presence of these chemicals in the body is harmful and will undermine the whole idea of homeostasis.

Protein

According to Dr. Sebi, the concept of protein interferes significantly with the natural functioning of the body. Instead, Dr. Sebi focuses on minerals and other elements. One prominent mineral that was the focus of Dr. Sebi in enjoying good health is nitrogen.

This is because nitrogen stands as the building block of your enzymes and muscles. They need continuous assimilation of nitrogen compounds to retain the best health. However, under the western diet, the belief is that you need meat to get this nitrogen.

The reality is that this is not the case. You can get these necessary nitrogen compounds in plants as well. Furthermore, these nitrogenous compounds also have large molecules of the necessary amino acids that your body needs. Unfortunately, like you, most people have forgotten that they can also get protein from plants. Even worse, there is some belief that animal protein is complete and more potent than plant protein.

However, this is not the case. Plant protein is just as complete and potent as animal protein. The good news is that it then excludes the various chronic diseases associated with meat and animal protein. For instance, a study that sought to support animal protein also realized that it supported cancerous cells' accelerated growth.

It becomes quite evident that the way forward for good health is plant proteins. It allows you to support good health without worries about the problems and health issues associated with animal protein.

Examples of plant protein foods include grains, nuts, seeds, and legumes. You can also rely on fruit and vegetables. However, keep in mind that they do not have as much concentration of nitrogen compounds as the earlier stated options.

Milk

While western milk is far from healthy for you, that does not mean you need to deny yourself of milk. This is because you can easily make your milk for yourself. We will discuss the recipe to achieve this subsequently.

Regardless, keep in mind that coconut milk, hemp-seed milk, and walnut milk are great options that should help start your healing process.

Energy

There is no doubt that the body needs the energy to perform its necessary body functions. This is why carbohydrates are a significant aspect of a healthy meal. However, when we say carbohydrates, we do not mean consuming carbohydrates the western diet way.

There are other safe means through which you can provide your body with adequate energy to carry out its necessary functions. You can achieve this through fruits. In case you didn't know, fruits have a high concentration of carbohydrates that can satisfy the body's needs.

So, rather than processed foods for carbohydrates, you can now rely on fresh fruits. You get the necessary carbohydrates, and you do not need to worry about cancer-causing preservatives and additives.

Examples of fruit options that can get the job done include bananas, apples, cantaloupe, and berries. We will discuss other options later.

Cleansing

On your road to healing, you need to cleanse your body. You can achieve this with the use of vegetables. This is thanks to its high micronutrient components. This is also thanks to the presence of vitamins, phytonutrients, fiber, and minerals in vegetables. They help you cleanse your digestive tract and boost your body's immune system.

Examples of vegetable options that you can rely on for cleansing include amaranth greens (callaloo), chayote (Mexican squash), avocado, bell peppers, and cucumber. We will discuss other options later.

Oils

While oil is necessary within the body, its use must be reduced to the barest minimum. This is because it is not a whole food. In turn, its excessive use can cause inflammation, damage the arteries, and promote the emergence of diabetes within the body.

So, while you can use some oils such as grape-seed oil, hemp-seed oil, sesame oil, olive oil, and coconut oil, reduce their use to the barest minimum. Ensure that you do not cook with them as high heat destroys their integrity.

Seasonings

If you must use seasonings, you must transition from the western idea of seasoning to ensure that you enjoy the best health. Examples of seasoning options that you can use include: achiote, basil, cayenne (African bird pepper), bay leaf, cilantro, habanero, coriander, dill, and onion powder. We will discuss other options later.

Herbal Teas

Tea is a popular aspect of the western diet. However, as you have now learned, this is far from the healthiest option, especially where you combine caffeine and milk. To transition to the alkaline-based diet, you must move to herbal teas.

These various herbal teas do not have caffeine in them. Even better, they have various phytonutrients that boost your immune system. So, you do not lose anything health-wise, but you gain something. We will discuss the various options later.

Sugars

You need to ensure that your intake of sugar is highly minimized. This is even more important where this sugar contains additives. As such, where you intend to consume sugar, the best bet is to consume date sugar. It represents the healthiest option available.

This is because when you consume date sugar, all you are consuming is grounded dates. It retains all its nutrients except for water. You can also consume pure agave syrup, which comes from cactus.

While it was once okay to consume maple syrup and grade B maple syrup, this is no longer the case. This is because most producers of this syrup use formaldehyde, which is toxic to the body.

Herbs and the healing process

Another important element of the healing process is the use of herbs. In fact, herbs are a core component of healing. This is because it comes with a high concentration of phytonutrients and nutrients. This composition then functions to help the body combat various bacteria and diseases. Even more, it also functions to clean the body of all harmful toxins within the body.

However, you must understand that herbs are best suitable for an environment where that is alkaline. That is, herbs are more effective when you combine them with alkaline foods. On the other hand, you will only be limiting their effectiveness when you eat acidic foods. This is because acidic foods are counterproductive to the herbs and will only undermine their efficacy.

Now, when it comes to herbs, there are various steps you need to understand. While herbs are effective, they are only functional where you have a suitable environment for them. In fact, this is the basis of the earlier instruction to combine herbs with an alkaline diet.

So, what are these steps and things that you need to understand?

Firstly, you need to understand the different types of herbs before you apply them to your healing. This is because various herbs exist, and they are suitable for a wide range of issues. For instance, herb A might be best suitable for disease B. In turn, when you apply that same herb A to disease C, you might not get the desired result. So, ensure that you understand the various types of herbs and the distinct function that they all perform.

Next, you need to choose between self-made herbs and commercial herbs. Typically, you can opt for a commercial herb, which is much easier. However, the downside to this option is that such an herb might not have been brewed under the best conditions. In turn, it might not have the best quality that you need to get the desired results. You cannot always ascertain that the quality advertised is what you are getting.

On the other hand, growing your own herbs comes with much more stress and responsibility. However, the great news is that you do not need to worry about the quality of the herbs where you do it rightly. In turn, you can count on getting the result that you desire from the herb.

All you need to do is get your seeds from wild crafted plants. You can always transplant these wild crafted to your home then grow under natural conditions. This means that you avoid the use of synthetic fertilizers on the grounds. These plants will grow without needing any form of human intervention. As such, you can be sure of their potency and their effectiveness. However, you can always use natural fertilizers such as manure.

You can also purchase bulk herbs if you do not want to harvest them. This is better than the commercial option. This is because it allows you to get insight into what you are purchasing. Precisely, with bulk herbs, you can thoroughly investigate them to confirm their quality.

Now, note that with bulk herbs, they can either come as powdered or whole herbs. It would be best for you to opt for whole herbs to ensure that you can ascertain their quality.

Harvesting the herbs

After planting these herbs, the next step is to harvest these herbs. You must keep in mind that these herbs have various components such as the flower, buds, leaves, and roots. These various components perform various functions and have different potency. As such, you must be sure to harvest all parts.

However, note that you will need to harvest these different components at different times. This is because they are more potent at different times.

Roots

It would be best if you harvested your medicinal roots around early spring. You can also do this in early fall. This is because the herb has its vitality stored in its roots at this period.

Leaves

By spring and summer, you will witness the movement of nutrients and energy from the roots to the leaves. As such, this is the best time for you to harvest them. However, you will want to make sure that you harvest these leaves before the flowers and seeds emerge.

This is because the nutrients and energy remain in the leaves. Once the flower begins to emerge, energy is diverted to support the flowers. So, be sure to pick the leaves before this occurs.

Also, note that you should only pick strong and mature leaves. You also want to go for options with no damage from insects and those with vibrant colors.

Flowers

You can also pick your flowers by spring and summer. However, the best period is just before the flowers open up. This is because there is a buildup of energy that has neither declined nor dissipated.

Drying Your Leaves

There are cases where you do not intend to use your leaves immediately after you harvest them. In such a case, you will need to dry the leaves to ensure that you can retain the leaves' nutrients.

You can use either the traditional process of drying or a dehydrator. In the case of the traditional process, you want to dry under room conditions. So, avoid direct contact with sunlight, which will compromise the herb's quality. Similarly, you do not want a humid area as this will limit the leaves' capacity to dry.

When you use a dehydrator, ensure that the temperature is a minimum of 90 degrees and does not exceed 105 degrees Fahrenheit. This way, the quality of the leaves does not get compromised.

Storing Herbs

You can then store the herbs in airtight glass jars to keep them in good condition. Ensure that the leaves are well dried before you store them. This is also the case with bulk herbs. Then, keep the jar in a cool, dry, and dark place. This way, you can retain the medical capacity of the herbs for a longer duration.

Making Herbs

Getting the herbs is only one part of the healing process. In fact, it is merely the preparatory process. You will need to make the herbs that you will ingest into your body. There are various ways through which you can achieve this.

You can always break down your herbs into smaller parts. Alternatively, you can always maximize other extraction methods to get the chemical compounds that you need out of them. However, note that in cases where you use an extraction method, you will lose the fiber.

No doubt, you will enjoy some advantages. For instance, you will get the chemical compounds faster into the blood through extraction. This is because your body does not have to worry about breaking down the fiber. Still, it is not the best bet. As such, it would be best for you to use the herbs as a whole.

All you will need to do is grind the herbs into smaller pieces. This way, the body can maximize the components and nutrients fully. Similarly, you want to ensure that you do not consume the leaves as large pieces. This is because it will make it difficult for the body to break down the herbs easily.

So, ensure you break the leaves down into smaller pieces. You will want to chew them properly where you do not grind them. Regardless, your best bet will be to grind the herbs. It comes with a wide range of positives for your digestive systems. In turn, you can extract the nutrients and phytonutrients that you need faster.

Extraction

In some cases, you must extract the chemical compounds from the herbs. This is useful for some specific types of herbs. There are two major methods through which you can achieve extraction. They are infusion and decoctions.

Infusion

This is a process through which you get an herb's medicinal properties by boiling it in water. This can be by boiling the leaves, flowers, seeds, or buds of the plant. This is an option that you can apply to the softer plants part.

By boiling them, you get through their cell wall and gain the necessary nutrients that you need. Keep in mind that this is quite popular today. Here is a guide on how to perform an infusion.

- Get the herbs your need, usually a tablespoon of dried herbs and one and half of a fresh herb

- Next, boil eight ounces the remove it from the fire

- Now, put the herb inside the water and allows it to steep between 30 and 45 minutes. You will find the water getting thicker with the more time the herb spends inside the water

- You can now drain the water and drink it Now, note that one tablespoon needs eight ounces of water. So, you can always increase the tablespoon and water appropriately.

Decoction

The second extraction method involves decoction. This is like an infusion. However, in this case, you use the plant's tougher parts. For instance, this will include parts like the twig, root, and bark.

Now, you will need to do more than just boil them. This is because they have a stronger cell wall that the water will not be enough to penetrate. So, after boiling, you want to go one more by simmering the herb. This will ensure that you can get the chemical compounds out better.

Here is a guide on how to perform an infusion.

- Get the herbs your need, usually a tablespoon of dried herbs and one and half of a fresh herb

- Next, boil eight ounces

- Now, put the herb inside the water and allows it to simmer for around 30 minutes. At this point, rather than put off the fire, you will only reduce it

- You can now allow the water to cool off

- You can then add it to a mason jar and drink it.

Again, one tablespoon needs eight ounces of water. So, you can always increase the tablespoon and water appropriately.

Grinding

As we stated, taking whole herbs is the best bet if you want to get the best result from your herbs. However, you cannot consume the leaves or flowers in large pieces. Then, it would be impossible for your body to process them appropriately and derive the necessary nutrients.

One way you can solve this is through grinding. It allows you to break down the leaves or plant parts into fine particles. This way, when you consume them, they can easily get to work in your body.

Now, you can always use a coffee grinder for the soft plant parts to get them into smaller particles that you can consume. Plant parts that fall under this category include the leaves, flowers, seeds, and buds.

On the other hand, for thick plant parts such as the root, bark, or twig, this will not work. As such, an industrial grinder becomes necessary. They have more power to get the job done.

Once you complete this, you can always put it in a capsule. All you need to do is get an encapsulation kit. With it, your task becomes pretty easy.

Dosages

Remember that upon the completion of such grinding and encapsulation, you will need to take them in the right dosage. While this is not as serious as you have in pharmaceutical medicine, you will still need to take it seriously.

Typically, the right dosage as an adult gets measured based on your weight. If you weigh 150 pounds, you will need around six grams of the capsule per day. With each capsule that you create, you will have around half a gram of the herb. In turn, you will need to take as many as 12 capsules each day.

Now, when it comes to children, you cannot apply the same dosage rule as adults. You will need to determine the appropriate dosage for them. In most cases, you will need what is known as Clarke's rule to archive this. The formula is expressed as follows:

Weight of the child (in lbs) x Adult dosage
———————————————————————————

150(Average weight of the child in lbs)

Combining Herbs

In some cases, we combine herbs to get the best results. For instance, we might combine more than one herbs for the same illness and simultaneously. Now, while there is no problem with this, you will need to be careful about your combination of herbs.

The general rule is that you can combine as many as four to five herbs to treat a specific issue. However, do not go higher than that. It would be best to ensure you keep it within this limit. This way, you do not have problems getting the right balance of dosage.

Dr. Sebi's Alkaline Medicinal Herbs

In the preceding section of this chapter, we have discussed in detail how to maximize herbs for your healing process as you move from the western diet to a healthier alkaline based diet.

We will now dive into various alkaline herbs that have been tested and trusted to produce positive results within the body. Keep in mind that the various herbs we will identify under this chapter have their chemical composition intact. That is, there has been no case of genetic modification of hybridization whatsoever.

In turn, they are useful as you seek to reverse various diseases within your body and heal yourself. Regardless, this list, which mirrors Dr. Sebi's discovery over his lifetime, is far from exhaustive. There are still various other herbs out there that might be useful.

However, we have placed a special focus here thanks to their completely natural state. Precisely, while some other herbs might offer various advantages to the body, they are not completely natural. In turn, they sometimes introduce various other compounds into the body, which can reduce the herbs' efficacy.

So, here are the popular options that can rely on as completely natural based on Dr. Sebi's recommendations.

Arnica

This herb has its origin in North America, and it gets used only as topical creams. It is a powerful antiseptic and anti-inflammatory herb. However, it is only to be externally utilized as it is dangerous to the body when ingested.

You can use it to treat various external wounds. You will find that it promotes fast tissue regeneration while relieving pains. You can also use it to treat sprains, headaches, bruises, and arthritis. Remember that this herb is only relevant for external use.

Batana Oil

This has its origin in Honduras, South and Central America. It comes from the Elaeis oleifera tree. The oil has great relevance thanks to its fatty acids constituent. It also has some relevant phytonutrients and nutrients.

You can apply this oil to provide strength to your hair. It will also aid oil growth while providing some natural coloring to the hair. You will find grey hair turning brown upon application of this oil.

Bladderwrack

This herb has its origin in the Atlantic Ocean, Baltic Sea, North Sea, and the Pacific Ocean. It is commercially used as an iodine supplement. This is thanks to its high concentration of iodine. Traditionally, this herb has seen its application to the treatment of oversized and underactive thyroid glands. It has also been used to treat iodine deficiency.

This is one rich herb as it also contains calcium, potassium, and magnesium. This is apart from the presence of other trace minerals within it. It also comes with a wide range of phytonutrients that ensures that the body enjoys considerable nutrients.

Even more, it comes with antioxidant benefits. This herb is also associated with a reduced risk of estrogendependent illness thanks to its antiestrogenic effects. It further lowers the cholesterol and lipid levels within the body.

Even more, bladderwrack ensures that your skin enjoys better elasticity while reducing its thickness and preventing the breakdown of skin enzymes. This herb is also believed to have displayed antitumor and antibacterial properties.

Blessed Thistle

This herb has its origin in the Mediterranean. It is typically consumed in 2 capsules of 390mg three times within a day. However, there are some limitations to its use. Precisely, pregnant women or nursing mothers will need to consult with health care professionals before their use.

It comes with significant health benefits. This herb has a high concentration of oxygen. In turn, it allows it to enjoy significant application to the increase of circulation within the body. It also aids better delivery of oxygen to your brain, which improves brain function and supports lung and heart function.

Similarly, it comes with bitter phytonutrients. This allows it to support gallbladder and liver function. It also stimulates the human's upper digestive tract. This makes it a great option to aid digestion while improving appetite.

That is not all that there is to this herb. It also comes with diuretic and antifungal properties. In turn, you can apply it to treat hormonal disorders that are associated with menstrual interference. It can also improve and enrich nursing mothers' milk flow thanks to its galactagogic capacity.

It also functions to aid intracellular cleansing. As such, you can apply to clean the body of acid, mucus, and toxins.

Blue Vervain

This herb has its origin in North America. It comes with a wide range of benefits, including a diuretic, antimalarial, antimicrobial, and anti-inflammatory properties. Over the years, it has seen its application in the treatment of menstrual cramps. It also helps to increase milk production among nursing mothers.

It is also useful in the treatment of nervous disorders, anxiety, stress, and restlessness.

Other herbs include:

Burdock root: It is a diuretic, blood cleanser, antiinflammatory, antioxidant, antifungus, anticancer, antiviral, and antibacterial herb.

Cascara sagrada: It contains emodin, which has antiviral and anticancer properties.

Chaparral: It has antimicrobial and antibacterial, antitumor and anticancer, and antiulcerogenic and antiinflammatory properties.

Cocolmeca: It has anti-inflammatory, antiulcer, antioxidant, anticancer, diaphoretic, and diuretic properties.

Contribo: It is relevant in traditional medicine for arthritis and edema. It also aids the stimulation of your immune system while aiding white blood cell production.

Damiana: It has anti-anxiety and anti-aromatase properties.

Eyebright: It has anti-inflammatory and antiseptic properties. It is relevant in the treatment of blepharitis and conjunctivitis bacterial eye infections.

Guaco: It has anti-inflammatory, anti-allergic, and bronchodilator properties.

Huereque: It has hypoglycemic, antiobesity, and antimicrobial properties. It is relevant in traditional medicine to reduce blood sugar levels. It also aids the treatment of diabetes and aids weight loss. It can also help in the cleansing of the pancreas.

Hombre grande: It has antifungal, antiulcer, antimalarial, anticancer, and insecticide properties.

Hops: It has anticancer, anti-inflammatory, and antibacterial properties.

Hydrangea Root: It has anti-inflammatory, antiseptic, antiparasitic, lithotrophic, and autoimmune properties.

Lavender: It has anti-insomnia, anticonvulsant, antifungal, antibacterial, antispasmodic, anti-anxiety, analgesic, anti-inflammatory, and antidepressant properties.

Conclusion

Again, your choice of food plays an important role in your health condition. This is why you need to prioritize a healthy diet. Unfortunately, you cannot get this with the western diet. This is thanks to the mainstay presence yes preservatives and additives. There are also meat and dairy products, all of which contribute negatively to the body system.

In turn, it becomes necessary to transition from the western diet to a safer and healthy diet. In this case, the alkaline plant-based diet becomes the ideal solution. As such, you must seek alkaline alternatives to the various western diet. Only then can you maintain good health.

Still, this is not all. Herbs play a significant role as you transition from the western diet to the alkaline diet. They ensure that you can enjoy various benefits while avoiding the issues associated with the western diet.

In the next chapter, we will discuss Dr. Sebi's top alkaline foods.

BONUS CHAPTER

TIPS TO OVERCOME THE DIFFICULTIES OF A NEW DIET LIFESTYLE

Introduction

Starting your journey through the healing process requires a healthy diet. However, after reading up on all that you need to do, there is still one problem. Starting that healthy diet and maintaining it, is easier said than done. In most cases, you will find people returning to their western diet in little or no time after claiming they have moved to an alkaline-based diet.

It starts with just a little carbonated drink. Then, there is sugar, and in time, you are back to where you started from, potatoes and corn. The reality is that after getting used to a particular way of eating over the years, switching to a new diet is far from easy. In fact, it is quite challenging for everyone.

This is because you will have to change what you are very comfortable with. You do not need to allow those difficulties to limit you in your journey towards healthy living. You do not need to struggle and be among those 80 percent that constantly relapses and go back to their old eating habits.

Why is it difficult to keep to a new diet lifestyle?

It is no longer news that almost everyone struggles with keeping up with a new diet lifestyle. What is news is why this happens. Note that this is extremely important as it allows you to determine the issue and develop applicable strategies that will help you cope.

So, why will you struggle to keep up with the alkaline diet?

1. A BELIEF THAT IT IS IMPOSSIBLE TO KEEP UP

The first reason why various individuals have found it quite difficult to keep up with the alkaline diet is the belief that it is impossible. Unfortunately, it is another reason why you will most likely be unable to keep up.

You need to know your mind has a significant role in maintaining a healthy diet. When you allow your mind to believe that the task ahead is impossible, your mind has no reason to continue. Then, in no time, you will find yourself relapsing.

2. ABSENCE OF GROUP HELP

It is easier to believe that the task is possible when you see others doing this. Your mind has a way of drawing strength from others.

Absence of interaction with others undergoing the same process makes it seem like a difficult task. In some cases, it leads back to reason one where you assume that it is impossible. Then, in no time, you find yourself relapsing.

3. ABSENCE OF CONNECTION WITH THE NEW DIET

It is not enough that you have heard that an alkaline diet is good for our health. It is also important for you to understand all about the alkaline diet. In turn, you can deeply understand why it is important and identify with the diet.

Unfortunately, in most cases, either because we are looking for a quick fix, we fail to do this. In turn, it becomes easier for us to relapse at the first sign of difficulty.

4. IDEA THAT YOU ARE AT A DISADVANTAGE

Another reason why we find it hard to stick with a new diet is the belief that it allows us to stand out. In most cases, we believe that this diet puts us at a disadvantage, thus, it becomes harder to stick to it. After all, no one loves to remain at a disadvantage.

Tips to overcome these difficulties

Now that you understand the reason for the difficulties, the next thing is to combat these difficulties. Here are some tips that will help you.

1. TAKE IT ONE STEP AT A TIME

One important aspect of keeping yourself in line with a new diet is taking it one step at a time. It is extremely important that you go very easy on yourself. This is because it makes your task easier.

You will need to remember that in most cases, you will not see results in a day. Worse, trying to do this might make you push yourself beyond your limits. In turn, you find it impossible to cope with the new diet.

However, by taking it one step at a time, you can gradually ease yourself into the diet. You avoid unnecessary pressure that might result in a clawback. You get accustomed to the diet and build your body's acceptance of such a diet.

Starting small is the key! You could start by making yourself a green smoothie in the morning before starting your day, a leafy green salad for lunch. Day by day add more alkaline rich dishes to your meal plan and in time you will be where you want to be. You are still on your first day, and in no time, you are celebrating your first year maintaining the alkaline diet.

So, remember that this is a process. You do not need to be perfect in the first week. All you need to do is ensure that you record improvement. Even when you do not record any improvement in a week, it is not the end of the world. Just be better the next week.

2. SEEK GROUP HELP

As we stated earlier, thinking you are alone makes things harder. However, by seeing others go through the same process daily, you are encouraged to do the same yourself. For instance, a study shows that partners of those in a weight loss program usually lose weight. However, they are usually not on the program.

That shows the effect of groups within our lives. So, find your tribe or group. They will help you make sense of the whole process. They will provide more reasons why you can also do it. This reassurance is sure to go a long way in helping you cope.

In some cases, it can be just one person. It is more of an accountability partner that allows you to understand that you are not alone. Try getting your household members to support you with your journey.

3. IDENTIFY WITH THE DIET

You will need to want to do it if you will eventually pull through. If there is no reason to pull through, then you most likely will not pull through. So, be sure to ensure that you know why you are doing it.

One way to achieve this is by understanding the diet and how it can help you. With more understanding, you get more interested, and with more interest, it becomes easier for you. It is also great to have more than one reasons why you are doing it. They will serve as durable support pillars for you.

Conclusion

While it might appear difficult to stick with a new diet, it does not have to be the case. There are various actions that you can help yourself with. One prominent way to do this is by finding why you are interested. That is what motivate you to keep with this new diet. By having this motivating factor, you can keep yourself going.

BOOK 3

Dr. SEBI

A Plant-Based, Mucusless Diet: How to reverse depression and bloating by cleansing and healing your gut problems and revitalize your body

AMBER FLOREY

INTRODUCTION

Your body is your Temple and we all know that we need to keep it as healthy as possible. Even when we believe we are doing our best to keep our bodies in good health, its vitality tends to diminish through external obstructions. When we are looking to improve our overall health, it is important to look into what causes this obstruction to live a healthy life. Our lifestyles have a great impact on our well-being, and of course, there are many factors that come into play. The two main factors being food and exercise. A plant-based diet is a way to good health, as it eliminates some causative factors of disease.

It is a common fact that animal products like meat acidify the human body; as a response, the body produces mucus to protect itself from the acids. This mucus interrupts the flow of energy and builds up waste in the body. If you want to achieve radiant and dynamic health, you need to avoid mucus-forming foods and wholly embrace plantbased diets.

Animal-based foods and their negative effects on your body

Did you know that almost all celebrated foods that we eat today are harming us? Like most of the people around the world today, you may consume twice the amount of proteins than you should. This is particularly dangerous for your body, future, and the environment as well.

Consuming animal-based products, such as meat, eggs, or other dairy-based products, only increases your chances of developing cardiovascular issues, high cholesterol, diabetes, obesity, and heart diseases. Out of all these, heart diseases are the most primary cause of death for people around the world. But, there is one way to protect yourself – switch to a plant-based diet, which will significantly reduce the chances of you developing heart problems by at least 20%.

When you drink milk, it means that you are also consuming the sex hormones that are injected into cows to hasten their growth. According to studies, it has been found that these hormones can increase the chances of cancer, a disease that 41% of people will be diagnosed with during their lifetime. In fact, the President's Cancer Panel of America has named cancer as the 'second-leading cause of death' in the country. After you switch to a plantbased or vegan diet, the risk of cancer falls by 34%.

Animal protein, which is very similar to human protein, can set off the auto-immune process. Hence, it can lead to multiple sclerosis and Type 1 diabetes, which can also be linked to the consumption of cow's milk.

Animal-based diets can cause macular degeneration, cataracts, and Alzheimer's. Animal proteins form highlyreactive free radicals. On the other hand, plants are often filled with antioxidants, which prevent these types of health problems.

Sushi is something that is an acquired taste. If you love to eat Sushi (raw fish) then there is a high probability that you are eating mercury – the same thing that drives the Hatter from 'Alice in Wonderland' mad. The "mad Hatter disease" is formally known as Erethism, which is a neurological disease that comes from mercury poisoning. In fact, the Mad Hatter from Alice in Wonderland got the disease through his job, mercury used to be used in the process of hat making and that's where the term "Mad Hatter disease" came from. Symptoms of this disease include depression, memory loss, mood swing and irritability. While it will definitely not scatter your brains, your future generation will have the potential to develop a lack of motor skills and learning disabilities. Sushi is just one example of many foods that contain mercury; there are a lot of other types of meat products that are filled with toxins too.

If you live near livestock, there are chances that you may suffer from the consequences of air pollutants, such as hay and animal feed. All the effects of the pollution will manifest in diseases like asthma or bronchitis, the former of which is a fast-growing ailment around the world.

Additionally, you are at risk of getting diseases like salmonella and ringworm. This is because factory farms store the blood and feces in ponds or use them as manure to spread across the field, which can contaminate the groundwater. Irrigation and rain then transport the pathogens from these water sources to water meant for human consumption.

Since most factory farms make use of a majority of antibiotic supply on livestock, bacterial strains can mutate bugs, which then becomes almost impossible to remove with antibiotics. This can cause outbreaks of lethal and terrifying diseases and outbreaks.

For instance, a certain superbug bacterium killed more people in America than AIDS. If these bacteria become immune to antibiotics, medical experts and doctors will have a more difficult time to look for vaccinations and cures in the future.

If you tally all these cases like toxin intake, high cholesterol, strokes, bronchitis, hormonal disruptions, diabetes, obesity, and superbugs, then you have a serious problem on your hands.

According to experts, every morsel of meat that you eat is like a slap in the face of a hungry child. Indeed, the meat industry's unending pursue of resources has resulted in shameless plundering of energy, land, water, and other global reserves in magnitude far more than just the production.

Let us take a look at one example. When you are turning animals into commodities, you have to invest a lot of resources like land space, water, etc. The resources used are so much that just a single person going vegan will provide enough water for hundreds of people.

People who eat meat and other animal-based products are contributing to destroying the planet, instead of feeding it. Animal agriculture produces negative greenhouse gases like methane, which can lead to climatic changes. For example, you will have to feed incredible amounts of food to your cows, if you want to keep up with the demand for meat. However, this also leads to more waste. Since wastes give off methane gases, it contributes to ozone depletion by trapping the heat in the atmosphere.

The demand for animal-based products has turned California valley-water supplies into poisonous wells, the pig-meat factories in China to dog-meat facilities, and the rainforests in Latin America into dried-out grasslands.

This particular industry wants you to believe that you cannot survive without any animal-based products.

However, it will destroy your terrestrial home, the health of your families, and your medical arsenal.

It is also about the human body. Judging by looking at the physiology and anatomy derived from vegetarian primates, humans are not equipped to process meat and other animal-based products. You will find a lot of epidemiological and experimental studies that will tell you why animal-based protein is harmful to the human body.

For instance, animal protein is important for some carcinogens that are incorporated in the human DNA, which causes different forms of cancer. Proteins derived from plants do not have this capability. Hence, if you follow a plant-based diet religiously, you will not develop cancer.

From a humanitarian perspective, you should also know that the animals are not fed properly. Most of these farmraised animals are fed bottom-of-the-barrel feed, which is absolutely not natural for them.

Apart from leaving the animals completely unsatisfied, it also ruins their biological makeup. Most of them are starved of nutrients that are needed for healthy growth because of this unnatural diet. Apart from affecting the well-being of the animal, the meat products are not up to the standard quality, which affects the well-being of meat consumers.

Wrong thinking

Some people argue that eating animals could be classified as morally wrong. If you think about it, we are taught to detach ourselves from the process of "killing an animal". Most people pick up the clean packaged meat out of the fridge section of a supermarket and think nothing of it, but at the same time could not even contemplate eating an animal that had been killed in front of their eyes, with blood, screaming and all. What is the difference? Your supermarket bagged up "piece of meat" was once that sweet living creature. If we can live without consuming meat, then why do this to animals? Let's accept that even animals have the right to live and raising animals for the purpose of killing and eating them is morally wrong.

Additionally, consuming animal-based products is criticized for ecological and health grounds. However, we will concentrate on the wrongs done to animals in this section.

Violated interests

Even the most humane form of raising and killing animals for consumption will always violate the most basic interest of the animal – to continue living. Modern animal farms often violate a lot of key animal rights like:

- eating a natural diet

- leading a healthy life without external medications
- living a life without pain or fear

- living in their natural environment

- living in decent conditions

Modern agriculture means that most animal farms keep their animals in over-crowded dirty cages or stalls, where some animals are unable to even take a few steps throughout the day. Living a life they were not meant to live in un-natural conditions, eating food they were not made to eat. Pumped full of antibiotics and growth hormones, which does not only harm them, but us, the consumer too! They are even deprived of medical care and suffer tremendous pain.

In the case of human interests vs. animal rights, most humans do not think that animals need any rights. However, this is always up for debate. However, human interest in meat is classified as trivial, since humans do not require meat to survive.

CHAPTER 1

PLANT-BASED DIET

Now, let us firstly begin with understanding what a plantbased diet is before going any further.

What is a plant-based diet?

Simply put, a plant-based diet is any diet that focuses more on types of foods that come from plant sources, which include nuts, legumes, pulses, grains, vegetables, fruit, and meat substitutes like soy products.

Most people have different interpretations of what a typical 'plant-based' diet looks like. Some may include small portions of animal-based products like fish and meat; however, they will mainly focus on vegetarian options. This is known as a flexitarian or semi-vegetarian diet.

Then, there are diets that may completely cut out meat, except for fish; this is known as a pescatarian diet. Next, we have people who include eggs and dairy products in their meals, who are known as vegetarians. Lastly, we have vegans who have eliminated all animal-based products from their diets, like gelatin, honey, eggs, and dairy.

People who follow plant-based diets end up consuming a wide range of pulses, vegetables, and fruits, which makes it easy to meet their five-a-day target. Thanks to this diet, they have healthy levels of minerals, vitamins, and fiber in their system that are present in vegetables and fruits, like potassium, Vitamin C, folate, etc.

However, it should also be remembered that a 'plant-based diet' does not automatically mean 'healthy,' especially if you consume a lot of packaged and processed food items. Some types of foods that come under these categories include certain vegetable fats, white flour, refined sugar, etc.

Plant-based diets, including vegan options, are considered very healthy if you consume them to the required nutritional level and balance. When you follow them consistently, a diet that consists of seeds, nuts, legumes, vegetables, fruits, and whole grains will provide you with a wide range of health benefits. For instance, you will be protected against certain types of cancers like breast and prostate cancer. There will be a reduced incidence of chronic diseases like heart ailments and Type-2 diabetes.

Also, your cholesterol levels and body mass index (BMI) will be lowered.

Similar to other types of diets you will come across today, the health benefits will mostly depend on the nutritional adequacy and quality of the diet. This means that you will have to replace white carbohydrates with whole grains and avoid sweetened and sugary beverages. Also, you will have to direct your attention to plant-based fats and proteins, like those found in seeds and nuts.

When you are following a plant-based diet, there are some key areas where you need to direct your attention. For example, you need to include nutrients like minerals, vitamins, Vitamin B-12, and proteins for healthy bone management.

Certain nutrients cannot be found in plant-based foods, like omega-3 fatty acids and Vitamins B12 and D. Hence, you will have to source them from fortified food items like cereals, spreads, and fortified plant milk.

Alternatively, you can also opt for supplements for supporting your nutritional intake. However, it is important that you have a serious talk about the subject with your doctor. If you plan on following this diet, you will have to plan your meals more carefully. It will be helpful if you arm yourself with some dietary information.

Benefits of a plant-based diet

For many years now, food scientists and registered dieticians have debated about the perks of an all-plant diet and avoiding animal-based products. However, people today are opting more for plant-based diets. This is because of the several advantages this diet has to offer.

According to experts, it has been said that a plant-based diet reduces the environmental impact of humans. In fact, celebrities like Tom Brady and Beyonce have embraced this type of diet. Here are some well-known benefits of a plant-based diet:

Lowers blood pressure

Hypertension or blood pressure increases the risk of several health problems like Type-2 diabetes, stroke, or heart diseases. Thankfully, the food that you eat can make all the difference. According to research, it has been found that a plant-based diet can easily reduce your blood pressure, which will reduce your risk of developing these health problems.

Another study concluded that people who consumed an all-vegetarian diet had lower blood pressure than those that followed an omnivorous diet, which included both meat and plants. Also, vegetarians had 34% lower chances of developing hypertension than meat-eaters.

Keeps the heart healthier

It is known that meat contains saturated fats, which contribute to heart problems when consumed in excess. Hence, eating plant-based foods and cutting back on meat is actually doing your heart a favor. Studies have proven that a plant-based diet will reduce the risk of developing cardiovascular diseases by 16%.

However, it is not only about cutting down on meat. You need to ensure that the plant-based foods you eat are very healthy. This means that you will have to load up on healthy oils (like olive oil), vegetables, fruits, legumes, and whole grains, rather than packed or processed vegetarian foods like sugary beverages and refined grains, which will only increase the risk of developing heart problems.

Prevent Type-2 diabetes

The link between a proper diet and Type-2 diabetes is well-known. Weight is considered a major factor since fatty tissue will make the cells more insulin-resistant. But, how do you know which diet is the best to avoid Type-2 diabetes? According to years of research, it has been concluded that by swapping to a plant-based diet you reduce your risk of developing Type-2 diabetes by 34%.

This is mostly because plants contain lower amounts of saturated fats than animal-based products. Saturated fats raise cholesterol levels and the risk of developing Type-2 diabetes increases as well. Another study states that Type2 diabetes is 7% higher in people that eat meat.

Helps in weight loss

After you change from animal-based products to plantbased products, the risk of obesity decreases significantly. Vegans and vegetarians mostly weigh less, even if that is not the primary goal here. The overall aim is to nourish the cells and tissues of the body to improve health outcomes; however, weight loss may be a by-product of reducing certain types of foods and replacing them. It has been studied that the difference in the BMI of vegans/ vegetarians and meat-eaters is quite significant – for the latter, it is 28.8 and 23.6 for the former.

Eating more plant-based products will help you lose a tremendous amount of weight. People that follow a plantbased and whole-food diet for a year can easily drop about 9.25-lbs. This is because vegetables and whole grains have a lower glycemic index, which means they get digested slowly. Additionally, fruits contain fiber and antioxidants that prolong the feeling of fullness. If weight-loss is your goal, then it is very important to eat healthy plant-based foods.

Helps live longer

All the above-mentioned benefits of a plant-based diet have one thing in common – help you live longer. Studies have concluded that plant-based diets lower the mortality rate by 25%. Also, your body's immunity system improves by 5% if you consume healthy plant-based foods.

However, you need to ensure that the plant-based foods you eat are healthy. According to studies, less-healthy plant-based foods include white bread, cake, and soda – while they are indeed meat-free, they are considered unhealthy. On the other hand, fruits, vegetables, and whole grains are considered much healthier.

Decreases the risk of cancer

As we have seen above, plant-based diets have a lot of health benefits – but the question here is whether it can prevent cancer? According to scientists, the answer could very well be yes. According to their studies, the best way to prevent cancer is to consume cancer-protective nutrients like phytochemicals, minerals, vitamins, and fiber. All these nutrients can be found in seeds, nuts, vitamins, beans, whole grains, vegetables, and fruits.

Additionally, studies have concluded that these protective benefits are present in moderate quantities, which can lower the risk of some types of cancers by 10%. Most of these nutrients are found in plant foods and will promote a healthy weight and lifestyle.

Improves cholesterol

In the case of high cholesterol, all the fatty deposits are lodged in the blood, which can restrict the flow of blood and will eventually lead to heart disease, stroke, or heart attack. However, a healthy diet will help keep the cholesterol levels in check.

When you move from an animal-based diet to a plantbased one, you lower the 'bad' cholesterol (LDL) by 15%; you can further lower this number by 25% if you are a strict vegan.

Minimize the chances of a stroke

When you are overweight, you will have high blood pressure. In turn, this increases the risk of stroke. Additionally, some other factors that increase the chances of strokes or developing other types of heart diseases include the use of drugs, drinking, smoking, having high cholesterol levels, etc. Most of these risks can be removed from the equation by following a plant-based diet and following a healthy lifestyle.

If you did not know this previously, strokes are preventable. One of the best ways to minimize the risk of strokes is to increase the intake of vegetables and fruits. It has been studied that people that consume vegetables and fruits daily have a lower chance (21%) of a stroke than meat-eaters.

Common plant-based foods With their benefits

People that follow a plant-based diet avoid eating animals for health, ethical, and environmental reasons. Sadly, following a plant-based diet is not easy as some people are at higher risk of suffering from nutrient deficiencies. This scenario can turn out to be quite true if the diets are not well planned.

If you are new to a plant-based diet, it is important that you include fortified and whole foods. Here are some common plant-based items that should be a part of a healthy plant-based diet:

Vegetables and fruits

There are some plant-based food eaters, especially the new ones, which rely heavily on vegan junk food and mock meats to replace their favorite meat products. However, most of these items tend to be very unhealthy and highly processed.

Thankfully, there are several ways to replace these items with vegetables and fruits, which are rich in minerals and vitamins. For example, mashed bananas can be used in baking recipes, instead of eggs. You can also opt for banana ice cream, instead of dairy-based ice creams. All you need to do is blend a frozen banana until it is smooth; all you have to do next is add your preferred toppings.

If you miss the meaty texture, you can opt for mushrooms (especially Portobello or cremini) and eggplants. They are also very easy to grill. Alternatively, you can also opt for jackfruit instead of meat for savory dishes like barbeque sandwiches and stir-fries.

Cauliflower is a great choice to add to several types of recipes, like pizza crust. To increase the intake of calcium and iron, plant-based food eaters eat a lot of leafy greens like mustard greens, watercress, kale, spinach, and bok choy. Some other great options include blackcurrants, artichokes, turnip greens, and broccoli.

The bottom line is that vegetables and fruits are quite healthy and some can even be used as substitutes for some animal-based foods.

Foods rich in Choline

Choline is a nutrient that is important for your nervous system, brain, and liver. While our body is capable of producing it, the amount is very small. Hence, it is important that you get this nutrient from outside sources.

This nutrient can be found in a wide range of grains, legumes, nuts, vegetables, and fruits, plant foods like quinoa, broccoli, cauliflower, soymilk, and tofu include the highest amounts. Choline is important for the proper functioning of the human body.

During pregnancy, women require more choline every day. The increased risk of choline deficiency can be seen in post-menopausal women, heavy drinkers, and endurance athletes. Hence, plant-based food eaters that fall into these categories need to ensure that consume as much choline-rich food as they can.

Cereals, whole grains, and pseudo cereals

Cereals, whole grains, and pseudo cereals are considered the best sources of many types of nutrients like selenium, zinc, phosphorus, magnesium, Vitamin B, iron, fiber, and complex carbs. Some of the varieties are more nutritious than others, especially protein.

For example, each cooked cup (237-ml) of teff and spelt grains contain about 10-11-grams, which is a lot more than rice and wheat. Then, there are pseudo cereals like quinoa and amaranth that have 9-g of proteins per cooked cup. These two are also sources of rare complete protein in this category.

Fermented and sprouted plant foods

While they are quite nutritious, a lot of plant foods also
have different levels of anti-nutrients. Anti-nutrients are
substances that reduce your body's ability to absorb the
minerals and nutrients in these foods. Hence,
fermentation and sprouting are considered the best and
simplest methods to minimize the number of
antinutrients found in different plant-based foods.

With the help of these techniques, you will be able to
absorb more beneficial nutrients from plant foods to
boost your overall health and protein intake. Interestingly,
sprouting has been known to reduce a small percentage of
gluten found in certain types of grains.

On the other hand, fermented plant foods contain
probiotic bacteria, which improve the digestive health and
the immune function of your body. They also contain
Vitamin K2, which is a great choice for improving dental
health and bone, as well as reduce the risk of cancer and
heart disease.

You can try to ferment or sprout grains in your home. If
not, you can purchase them from your local stores; they
are mostly known by names like kombucha, kimchi,
pickles, sauerkraut, natto, miso, tempeh, etc.

Nutritional yeast

From the deactivated strain of the yeast Saccharomyces
cerevisiae, you get nutritional yeast. They are available in

the form of yellow flakes or powders in health food stores and supermarkets. A single ounce contains roughly 7-g of fiber and 14-g of protein. Additionally, nutritional yeast also contains Vitamin B12, manganese, copper, magnesium, and zinc.

Hence, fortified nutritional yeast can be the best way for plant-based dieters to get their daily dose of Vitamin B12. However, you also need to know that Vitamin B12 is light sensitive and may degrade if stored in clear plastic bags. Alternatively, you should never rely on non-fortified nutritional yeast for Vitamin B12.

Calcium-fortified yogurts and plant milk

Vegans and plant-based food dieters consume lesser amounts of calcium than meat-eaters and regular vegetarians, which do have a negative impact on their bone health. This is mostly because the daily calcium intake falls well below 525-mg per day.

For this reason, you need to consume calcium-fortified plant yogurts and plant milk and try to make them a part of your daily menu. If you also want to increase your protein intake on the way, look for plant yogurts and milk made from hemp or soy. Lower protein alternatives include oat milk, rice, almond, and coconut.

Mostly, calcium-fortified plant yogurts and milk also contain Vitamin D, a nutrient that helps in calcium absorption. Some brands also add Vitamin B12 separately.

If you want to reach your daily intake of Vitamin B12, Vitamin D, and calcium, always look for fortified plantbased milk and yogurt. You can add some sugar if you want; however, ensure that you keep it to a minimum.

Minimally processed meat substitutes like tofu

There are some minimally processed meat substitutes that are made from soybeans, like tempeh and tofu. Both items contain about 16-19-g proteins per 100-g portions. They are also great sources of calcium and iron.

Tofu is created by pressing soybean curds; it is known to be one of the most meat replacements since it can be scrambled, grilled, and sautéed. They are also good alternatives for eggs in recipes like quiches, frittatas, and omelets.

You can also make use of tempeh as meat replacements. It is made from fermented soybeans and is a popular replacement for fish, thanks to its distinctive flavor. However, you can also use it in many other types of dishes.

Additionally, the fermentation process will also reduce the number of anti-nutrients found in soybeans, which means your cells will absorb more nutrients from the tempeh dish. The fermentation process also contains small amounts of Vitamin B12, something that is normally found in animal-based products.

Another great alternative for meat is seitan, which provides 25-g of wheat protein per 100-g. This product is also rich in selenium and small concentrations of phosphorus, calcium, and iron. However, if you are gluten sensitive or have celiac disease, it is recommended that you avoid seitan, as it contains a high concentration of gluten.

All these options are great alternatives to heavily processed mock meats like vegan chicken fillets and vegan burgers, which contain a lot of additives and very few nutrients.
You can eat them once in a while.

Legumes

To avoid animal cruelty and exploitation, vegans avoid typical sources of proteins like eggs, fish, poultry, and meat. Therefore, you need to look to replace iron and protein sources with plant-based alternatives like legumes.

Some great options include peas, lentils, and beans, which contain about 10-20-g proteins per cup (cooked). They are also great sources of other health-promoting plant compounds like various antioxidants, zinc, manganese, folate, iron, slowly digested carbs, and fiber. Apart from these, legumes also contain small amounts of antinutrients, which reduce mineral absorption in the body.

The absorption of iron from plant-based food is at least 50 times lower than animal-based products. Similarly, zinc absorption is 35% lower in plant-based foods as compared to items that contain meat.

If you want to increase zinc and iron absorption, you may have to avoid eating legumes at the same time as foods that contain calcium. This is because calcium can hinder the absorption process. Instead, you can eat legumes with vegetables and fruits that are rich in Vitamin C to increase iron absorption.

Overall, it can be said that peas, lentils, beans, and other types of legumes are perfect animal-based food alternatives as they are rich in many different types of nutrients that are beneficial for the body. Additionally, you can also cook, ferment, or sprout the legumes so that they can be absorbed easily by the body.

CHAPTER 2

PHLEGM AND MUCUS

Since we are talking about a mucus less diet in this book, it would only make sense if we understand what the terms 'mucus' and 'phlegm' really mean, its causes and symptoms, etc.

What are phlegm and mucus?

The body keeps producing phlegm and mucus constantly to prevent the body's internal tissues from dehydrating and protect it from infections. While they are always at work, you will only notice these sticky substances when you fall sick.

Both phlegm and mucus work as a part of your immune system and trap external particles when you breathe in air through your nose. The human body produces approximately 1.5-l of phlegm and mucus each day – even more, when you are sick.

Both are made from salt, protein, enzymes, antibodies, and water. They carry the debris, dust, and dead cells from the nose and lungs.

Difference between phlegm and mucus

Phlegm and mucus are both produced in the body. However, there are some differences that you should know. To understand the difference between phlegm and mucus, we need to break this section into two parts:

What is mucus?

Mucus is a slippery, watery, and gelatinous fluid that is released by the mucous membranes in the body. It is often seen when you blow your nose during the cold.

Mucus filters out a lot of different irritants like allergens, smoke, bacteria, and dust. They contain enzymes and natural antibodies that help fight against infections and bacteria. Additionally, it also captures debris and toxins to protect your lungs when you are inhaling via your nose or mouth, and then passed out of the system. When you have a runny nose, you will see a mixture of water secretions and mucus from your nose.

What is mucus made of?

As mentioned above, mucus is mostly made of proteins, inorganic salts, and water. They are produced by the mucous membranes in the nose and keep the organs from drying out by acting as a moisturizing and protective layer.

What is phlegm?

Phlegm is also a type of mucus that is mostly seen in the lower airways like the lungs and throat; they are made to respond to inflammation. When you are sick, your lungs cough up phlegm and expel the mucus through your nose.

What is phlegm made of?

Similar to mucus, phlegm is naturally produced in the body and made of proteins, inorganic salts, and water. While they may serve the same purposes, phlegm is a bit thicker than mucus.

When something is wrong with your body, the consistency and color of the mucus and phlegm will offer you clues as to what is going on. However, you cannot count on color as an indication of a viral or bacterial infection.

Common causes of phlegm and mucus

Phlegm is mostly associated with conditions, disorders, and diseases of the respiratory system like the lungs, bronchial tubes, trachea (windpipe), throat, and nose. However, they can also be caused by conditions in the cardiovascular system (like congestive heart failure) and the upper digestive tract.

The symptoms of phlegm are mostly caused by viral or bacterial infections in the upper airways and lungs. If your lungs are healthy, they will be covered with a thin layer of phlegm. When threatened by foreign substances (like dust or smoke) and infectious germs, your lungs will produce more phlegm. The phlegm thickens and needs to be expelled from the lungs via coughing to keep the airways clear.

There are certain types of foods, like dairy products, as well as medication for blood pressure that can increase the symptoms of phlegm. While most of these causes are quite simple, there are some that are life threatening.

As for mucus, there are a lot of health conditions that can lead to excess production of mucus. Some of them include lung diseases (like COPD, cystic fibrosis, pneumonia, and chronic bronchitis), infections (like the common cold), asthma, allergies, and acid reflux.

If you are producing excess mucus, it can also be due to certain environmental and lifestyle factors like smoking, certain medications, high consumptions of fluids that lead to loss of fluid like alcohol, tea, and coffee, low consumption of water, and dry indoor environment.

When you are sick because of a respiratory infection, you will notice that your mucus is thick and darker than usual. Additionally, this mucus is also thicker than your regular mucus. This mucus can also be associated with different symptoms like flu and cold. When you are sick, the mucus may also appear to be yellow-green in color. Excessive mucus is not generally a medical problem; however, they tend to be a nuisance and an uncomfortable experience.

Symptoms

The symptoms of mucus appear when the membrane lining on the digestive and respiratory tracts produce more mucus than usual, as a response to an allergen or irritant. This results in diarrhea, breathing difficulties, and congestions.

Some symptoms of mucus, like nasal congestion and runny nose, are common because of viral infections like common cold and allergies. Fungal, viral, and bacterial infections can cause pneumonia, bronchitis, and sinusitis that can cause the symptoms of mucus in the respiratory system.

Mucus symptoms can accompany other symptoms, which will depend on the underlying condition, disorder, or disease. Symptoms affect the mucous membranes that may also involve other systems of the body. You will find a lot of symptoms that can affect the respiratory system like:

- Wheezing (whistling sound when you breathe)
- Sore throat
- Sneezing
- Shortness of breath
- Nasal congestion or runny nose
- Shortness of breath or rapid breathing (tachypnea)
- Coughing up green, light brown, or yellowcolored mucus
- Coughing gets severe

Phlegm contains mucus and also other substances like foreign particles (dust), pus, and dead cells. While you may not notice phlegm, you will if you suffer from respiratory infections like pneumonia. If you have other conditions or diseases (like asthma or cystic fibrosis), your body may produce different types of phlegm.

The abnormal symptoms of phlegm can be caused due to a wide range of health issues like obstructions in the airway, medication, trauma, allergy, inflammation, malignancy, and infections. Additionally, if you consume certain types of foods like dairy products, taking certain medications, exposure to smoke, etc., it can cause symptoms of phlegm. Some common symptoms of phlegm include:

- Watery eyes
- Throat symptoms like white patches, enlarged tonsils, dry throat, sore throat on the throat and tonsils
- Tender and swollen lymph nodes
- Sneezing
- Stuffy or runny nose, often with yellow and green phlegm discharge
- Loss of appetite and nausea
- Muscle aches
- Headaches
- Fever with or without sweats and chills
- Fatigue

- Coughs

What is a mucusless diet?

Professor Arnold Ehret, the German alternative health educator, and naturopath studied the value of a specific dietary intake when he was traveling through North Africa. Since the professor only consumed fruits, he got dramatic results one example was that he was able to cycle 800 miles. This way he was convinced that the food we consume dictates how healthy we are.

Professor Ehret's concept and theories on a mucusless diet are still considered controversial; however, they do have a lot of following from all around the world. This concept is that you need to consume food that does not produce mucus, like leafy green vegetables, nuts, and fruits. He went on to create a dietary definition based on these food groups, along with additional supplements via flushing the digestive system with water and fasting.

Ehret emphasized how the body functions to remove toxins from the body. If you understand this process, you can control your natural balance, which will provide you with great benefits, like weight loss and increased performance, without nutritional deficiency. This type of diet typically goes beyond normal vegetarianism and even veganism. In short, a mucusless diet focuses on the first and original human diet.

In short, you can say that a mucusless diet is a diet system that progressively and gradually moves away from foods that form mucus to those that do not. The mucus-forming food eventually decomposes into slimy substances in the body. You can take rice as an example. When you melt rice down, you will get a very sticky substance. As a result, this sticky substance is known as mucus. In fact, rice is also used as glue for bookbinders at times. Now, the question here is – why would you want to consume something that turns into something sticky?

Foods that worsen phlegm and mucus

There are a lot of different types of foods that are known to increase the production of mucus and phlegm. Here are some types of foods that can cause a buildup in mucus. If you want to avoid respiratory conditions like chronic obstructive pulmonary diseases, you should avoid these foods or eat them in moderation:

Put an end to bloating

For people suffering from excessive mucus and phlegm, bloating is caused by the increased pressure on the diaphragm, which also worsens the case of dyspnea – the feeling of breath shortage. Sadly, there are a lot of highly nutritious foods that can be the reason behind the bloating – particularly cruciferous vegetables like bok choy, cauliflower, Brussels sprouts, kale, cabbage, and broccoli, which are high in vitamins like A and C.

The good news here is that you can get these nutrients from other types of foods like sweet potatoes, squash, carrots, and citrus fruits.

Other types of foods like fried food, alcohol, fizzy soda, and sugary treats can cause excessive mucus and phlegm secretion, in particular, fried foods, which are high in fat, digests slowly and causes bloating.

Steer away from salt

Salt can cause mucus to retain, which leads to fluid buildup in the lungs. If you have a breathing problem, the production of excessive mucus and phlegm can make breathing quite difficult. While you do not have to completely remove salt from your diet, you need to choose food items that have lower than 140-mg sodium content.

Some types of foods that have excessive salt content include tacos, burritos, soups, cured meats and cold cuts, pizza, and bread. Instead, you can prepare your own meals with fresh ingredients like whole grains, vegetables, and fruits to avoid unnecessary salt. When you are cooking, you can also add alternatives like spices and salt-free seasonings.

Remove cured meats

Some types of foods that increase the production of mucus and phlegm like process luncheon meats, cold cuts, bacon, hot dogs, etc. According to research, it has been suggested that eating any type of food that contains nitrites and nitrates, which are mostly used in preserved meats, can have harmful effects on the lungs and can increase the production of mucus and phlegm.

Additionally, the high consumption of these meats increases the risk of lung diseases like COPD; when the symptoms of such diseases become severe, you may get hospitalized.

While it is not clear how processed meats increase mucus and phlegm production, it has been speculated by experts that nitrites and nitrates can also damage the tissues of your lungs. The high salt content also aids in fluid retention.

Avoid spicy foods

Most people tend to eat spicy food when they have a cold since it thins out the mucus and phlegm and makes it easier to expel. This is true in some aspects; additionally, the capsaicin found in chilies provides a desensitizing effect and can also help manage inflammation.

However, new studies have emerged that capsaicin can also stimulate the production of more mucus and phlegm than usual. While a spicy item may relieve you of the symptoms for some minutes, things will only get worse in the long run and delay your overall recovery period.

Watch out for caffeinated beverages and drinks

There are several types of caffeinated beverages and drinks like coffee, tea, and soft drinks that can increase the risk of dehydration. In turn, this also leads to increased production of mucus and phlegm. The only solution here is that you need to replace your caffeinated drinks with water to ensure that the mucus secretion is lubricated and thin. Additionally, it has also been found that desserts and chocolates contribute to the thickening of mucus and phlegm due to the caffeine's dehydrating effects in these food items.

Moderate dairy-product intake

Dairy products like yogurt, ice creams, cheese, and milk contain high-fat content. When you pair these products with typical Western foods like sweets, red meat, and refined grains, your body tends to produce more mucus and phlegm that increases lung difficulties like lower lung function etc.

Drinking the cow's milk produces the production of mucus and phlegm. While it is often disputed, milk increases the thickness of mucus and can prove to be very uncomfortable, especially when you have breathing problems.

Additionally, dairy products can also cause bloating in people that are lactose-sensitive, which makes breathing more difficult.

With that being said, dairy products contain a lot of different essential nutrients that are important for lung health, like selenium, magnesium, Vitamin A, and Vitamin D. Additionally, milk-based products are also high in calcium, which are beneficial for people that cannot consume enough daily calories due to lack of appetite.

Hence, you can incorporate plant-based milk products into your diet. For added information, you can get in touch with your doctor.

Avoid food allergens

If you are allergic to some types of foods, you will experience increased production of mucus and phlegm after eating the offending foods. There are several types of foods that trigger allergic reactions like soy products (tofu), gluten (pasta and bread), and dairy products. Some symptoms of food allergies include sneezing and nasal congestion. When you eliminate food allergens from your diet, you will decrease the production of mucus and phlegm. You need to test for food sensitivities to determine which foods you are allergic to.

Watch your entire diet

Apart from specific foods, the overall diet of a person can also contribute to increased secretion of phlegm and mucus. For instance, if your diet consists of starches (noodles and rice), red meat, and deep-fried foods can increase the production of phlegm and mucus, which can be bad for people with breathing difficulties.

While plant-based diets, like a Mediterranean diet that consists of healthy fats, whole grains, legumes, vegetables, and fruits have been found to decrease mucus and phlegm production and preserve lung function.

Natural foods and herbs that cleanse the body of mucus

When our body produces more mucus and phlegm that it normally should, we often think about the food we eat that may trigger this reaching. For most people, it may be allergenic foods like gluten (wheat), eggs, tree nuts, dairy products, and soy. For others, it may be a deficiency of certain minerals. Hence, your first line of business is to remove all these offending foods and add the following foods mentioned below:

Cucumbers

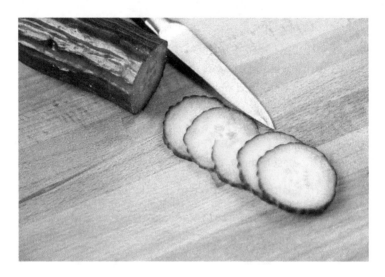

Cucumbers are known to be one of the top cleansing vegetables today. Also, they are rich in Vitamin C, potassium, and water. Vitamin C improves the immune health and the alkaline nature of the cucumber reduces the inflammation in the digestive tract and nourishes the gut lining, thereby improving the immune system further.

Onions

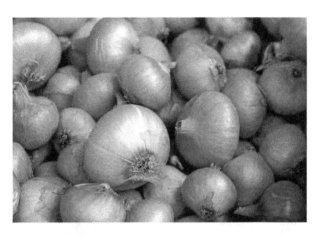

Onion is a pungent vegetable that is high in quercetin flavonoid that helps you that will improve respiratory function by acting as a natural antihistamine to respond against allergic responses and reduce inflammation. Onions are considered the most basic vegetables since they can be added to all types of cooked foods like stews and roasts or be chopped up to be added to salads. While your eyes may water white you cut through it, it definitely is filled with many health-boosting properties.

Broccoli

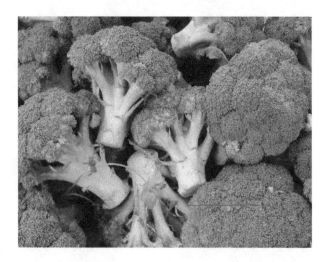

Broccoli is a vegetable that is packed with detoxification properties. It feeds the good bacteria and helps the waste move smoothly through the body.

Carrots

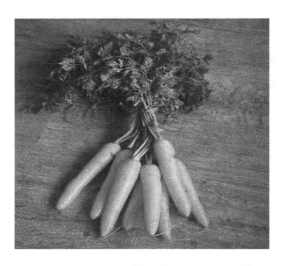

Carrots are tasty root vegetables that can nourish you on a cellular level. It contains high amounts of Vitamin A to improve the immune health, fiber, potassium (ultimate body cleanser), and Vitamin C. These root vegetables can be consumed raw or cooked as a tasty dinner side, instead of refined carbs and wheat pasta that can weaken good bacteria and enhance the production of mucus.

Pineapples

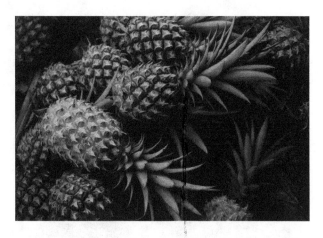

There are several fruits that can help solve the problem of excessive production of mucus in the body. Perhaps the best choice here is the pineapple. Pineapples contain proteolytic enzymes that break down proteins. It also has anti-inflammatory properties that will boost your immune function and open up your airways. Pineapples also contain bromelain that will improve the conditions of your sinus and reduce the production of mucus and swelling, thereby clearing the lower and upper respiratory tracts.

Grapefruit

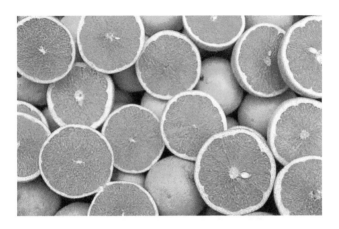

Grapefruit is a tart citrus fruit that is filled with cholesterol-fighting properties. Additionally, the high salicylic acid content will help you bring down the production of mucus and reduce inflammations that are often caused by allergies. The salicylic acid has the same anti-inflammatory properties as aspirin. Additionally, the high pH level will break down the proteins present in mucus, thereby thinning it down. Since the high tang of the fruit is not made for everyone, you can try mixing it with pineapple to combine the congestion-fighting abilities of both.

Vegetable oils

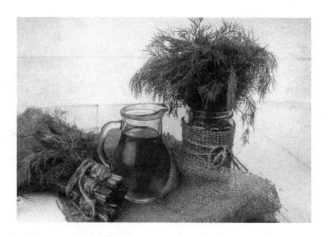

There are some vegetable oils that can ease your breathing and thin out the mucus in your chest. Some of these oils also restrict the growth of bacteria that may infect your respiratory tract. Some types of beneficial essential oils include oregano, thyme, tea tree, rosemary, peppermint, lemongrass, eucalyptus, cinnamon bark, and basil. Apart from consumption, these oils can also be used for inhalation or a vapor rubs.

Apple

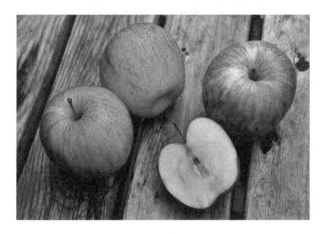

The fiber known as pectin and Vitamin C is found in apples. The nutrients are known to relieve the buildup of mucus in the body. The content of potassium adds to the abilities and can be eaten in several different ways. You can bake, juice, blend, or eat them raw. Alternatively, you can also use some pears and cinnamon to create a naturally sweet dessert. Or, you can use applesauce to replace sugar or butter to create a delicious batch of muffins.

Berries

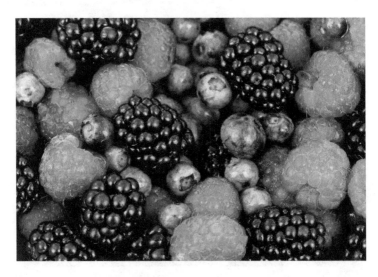

Berries are another option that is known to cleanse your body, especially your digestive tract. They are also great sources of antioxidants, potassium, and Vitamin C. All these nutrients will help you clean your blood and the fiber present will break down and remove the toxins to fight off infection and inflammation. You can use blueberries, blackberries, and raspberries in your next glass of smoothie, instead of sugary yogurts or artificial sugary sweeteners. They are naturally sweet and will add the perfect flavor, along with improving your immune health naturally and support cellular cleansing.

Pumpkin seeds

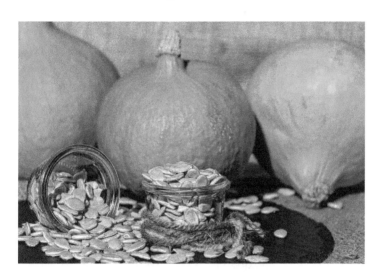

Pumpkin seeds are known to be one of the best sources of omega-3 fatty acids that can help you relieve inflammation. Additionally, it also contains magnesium that minimizes inflammation by relaxing the blood cells. Both of these nutrients can also be used to reduce the swellings of your sinuses caused by allergies, thereby allowing you to drain your mucus better and also prevent congestion. You can snack on them raw, bake them in some dishes, or sprinkle them on the salads. The antiinflammatory properties of the seeds will only provide you with a lot of health benefits.

Ginger

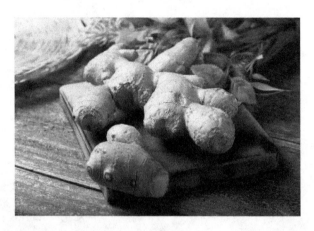

Ginger is known to reduce the production of mucus and break down toxins quickly, thanks to the many enzymatic benefits it has. Itis also packed with anti-inflammatory effects that will improve your immune system and reduces the production of mucus. It is recommended that you use fresh ginger; for more benefits, you can also use a bit of turmeric. You can try it in a vegetarian dish, tea, or can even be juiced to make some tasty smoothie.

Greens

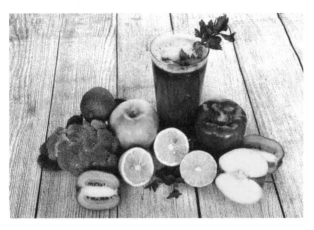

Greens are considered some of the best options to heal your body. They contain high amounts of Vitamin E, B, C, and A. Also, you will find potassium that supports the growth of your body on a cellular level. You can cook them at night, eat them the next day, or simply blend them in the morning in form of a smoothie. They reduce the production of mucus and toxins with ease. Additionally, the fiber can be used to feed the good bacteria while the high amount of chlorophyll improves blood health and support the immune system.

5 Plant-based recipes that provide relief from mucus

The food choices we make play a very important role when it comes to providing relief from mucus. These recipes will help you regulate and clear mucus. The juice is refreshing and will boost your immunity significantly.

Here are some delicious recipes that you can create with ease:

• Blood Orange, Carrot, and Ginger Smoothie

The blood orange, carrot, and ginger smoothie is a tasty and simple recipe that you can prepare quickly if you want some relief from mucus buildup and congestion. You can easily prepare a large pitcher of a gut-friendly and nutrient-dense decongestant to keep your mucus relief ready. The juice is sweet and a bit acidic as well. You will also love the fact that it is full of Vitamin C, which will boost your immunity, which makes it perfect for winters since this is the season when mucus starts building up in your respiratory tracts.

Prep time: Five minutes

Serves: Two

Ingredients:

- Pineapple (½ cup)

- Frozen banana (1)

- Knob grated fresh ginger (1, grated about 1-inch)

- Peeled blood orange cut into pieces (1)

- Peeled and chopped carrot (1)

- Coconut, cashew, or almond milk (2 cups, optional)

Instructions:

To create this recipe, you will only require a blender. You will have to juice about four-five blood oranges (depending on how you cut them). Next, you need to cut the ginger into small slices. Once done, you need to add the ginger, the orange juice, and a small amount of carrot into the blender.

Next, you just have to combine all the ingredients and blend it for a minute. To go a bit further, you can also add some coconut, cashew, or almond milk to boost the overall flavor and immunity-boosting properties. You can serve them in glasses once everything gets incorporated nicely. You can drink the smoothie immediately.

• Garlic and Onion Sunflower Seed Crackers

Garlic has been used to remedy cold and mucus buildup for thousands of years. This recipe is very easy to make and is filled with nutrients. This snack is perfect for people that suffer from allergies and can be dipped into your favorite sauce or soup to battle the buildup of mucus in your airways. ***Prep time:*** 10 minutes

Serves: Two

Ingredients:

- Water (½ cup)

- Onion powder (1 teaspoon)

- Garlic powder (½ teaspoon)

- Himalayan rock salt (1 teaspoon)

- Nutritional yeast flakes (1 teaspoon)

- Psyllium husks (1 teaspoon)

- Chia seeds (1 teaspoon)

- Flax seeds (¼ cup)

- Sunflower seeds (1 cup)

Instructions:

First, you need to start by preheating your oven to 180°C; alternatively, you can also fan force. Then, separate all the dry ingredients and add them to a processor. Keep blending them until they break down properly and get combined. To further blend the mixture, you can add some water.

On a lined baking tray, you have to spread out this mixture and smoothen it out with the help of a back of a table spoon or a silicone spatula. Spread this mixture nicely, with a thickness of 4-mm to create a single large cracker.

Bake the spread in the oven for 30 minutes or until the cracker turns golden brown. Once 20 minutes, remove the cracker and turn it upside down. Once the time is up, you can remove the cracker and let it cool down before you break it into different sizes and shapes. The cracker can then be stored in a glass jar for at least five days.

• Garlic Miso and Onion Soup

If you are looking for a vegan miso soup, there is nothing that can beat this garlic miso and onion soup. This is a very basic vegan/vegetarian recipe that can be cooked and served within a few minutes. This is originally a Japanese dish and many types of ingredients can be used to create this vegan miso soup.

This vegan recipe can also be made gluten-free, with the help of gluten-free miso. Alternatively, many grocery stores have different varieties of miso, like barley; this will allow you to make different varieties of soups. The garlic and the onions will help break down congestion and mucus in your chest and also help reduce your cough.

Prep time: 10 minutes

Serves: Six

Ingredients:

- Seaweed (1 tablespoon)
- Miso (½ cup)
- Silken tofu (1, diced)
- Sesame oil (1 teaspoon)

- Soy sauce (2 tablespoons)

- Garlic powder (¼ teaspoon)

- Garlic cloves (4, peeled and minced)

- Onion (½, peeled and minced)

- Scallions (3, chopped)

- Shiitake mushroom (½ cup, sliced)

- Water (5 cups)

Instructions:

The first thing you need to do is gather the ingredients and then heat water to a low simmer. Next, stir in the miso. Ensure that the water is not boiling, but just below the boiling point. Keep stirring the mixture until the miso gets fully dissolved in the pot.

Once the miso has mixed nicely, you can start adding the other ingredients. Make sure that the miso does not have any clumps when you are adding the other ingredients. Heat the mixture for some time, or unless the mushrooms and garlic get softened. Stir for another few minutes and the dish is ready to serve.

• Gingery Yellow Rice

If you are suffering from a cold and running nose, you can try digging your taste buds into some gingery yellow rice. Thanks to the amount of fresh ginger and inflammation resistant turmeric, this dish has a lot of health benefits. Turmeric also boosts your immune system, eases digestive discomforts, and heals your liver. However, you also need to be careful with the amount of turmeric you end up using, or else you will end up with a dish with a very bitter flavor. ***Prep time:*** 10 minutes

Serves: Two
Ingredients:

- Coconut milk (1 cup)
- Vegetable broth (2 cups)
- Sea salt (teaspoon)
- Ginger with juice (1 tablespoon, freshly-grated)
- Clover garlic (1, grated)
- Turmeric powder (1 tablespoon)
- Bay leaves (1 or 2)
- Lemongrass (2 stalks)
- White Jasmine Rice (2 cups)

Instructions:

Begin by rinsing the rice at least three times and then add it to your saucepan. Remove the root ends of the lemongrass stalks and then the dry top sections. With the help of your knife's handle, mash the root ends. Remove the layers of the lemongrass and tie them in knots. After that, add it to the rice.

Mix up all the remaining ingredients to the rice and stir it to mix it properly. Start the boiling process, then reduce the heat, and let the rice simmer for the next 15 minutes. Shake the pot for better mixing without removing the lid.

Shut down the heat and allow the rice to sit for another five minutes. All this while, do not remove the lid because the rice is getting its final steam and the excessive moisture is getting absorbed. Once it cools down, you can serve it hot.

• Spicy Sweetcorn and Onion Fritters

If you are looking for a crispy and delicious dish that can also help with mucus relief, you can try this particular dish. Apart from the heat that will help with congestion in your chest, it is also rich in onions. They make a perfect lunch and you will have a taste of deep-fried food without the requirement of deep-frying. The yogurt is dairy-free and will help you balance the taste of the vegan dish.

Prep time: 10 minutes

Serves: Two

Ingredients:

For the yogurt sauce

- Plain soy yogurt (½ cup)
- Lime (½, juiced)

- Fresh coriander (¼ cup, roughly chopped)

- Black pepper

For the fritters

- White onions (2, sliced into rings)

- Black pepper

- Chili flakes (¼ teaspoon)

- Water (½ cup)

- Light olive oil (2 tablespoons)

- White onion (1, medium, finely chopped)

- Corn flour (½ cup)

- Buckwheat flour (½ cup)

- Fresh coriander leaves (¼ cup, roughly chopped)

- Garlic clove (1, crushed)

- Sweet corn (1 ¾ and 2 ¾ tablespoons each)

Instructions:

To first make the fritters, you need to slice two onions and keep them aside. Next, place all the other ingredients in a bowl and mix them properly. Heat the light olive oil and add the onion rings to it, along with the mixture. The onion rings will prevent the batter from spilling out. Cook the entire mixture for not more than 15 minutes and keep turning them for an even cook.

For the yogurt, mix the combination of black pepper, coriander, lime juice, and soy yogurt until it becomes consistent. You can serve the fritters with the yogurt and add a slice of fresh lime for garnishing.

CHAPTER 3

SWITCHING TO A PLANT-BASED DIET

After hearing the truth about the meat industry, many people decide to go vegan. However, the transition may not be easy for all people. If you are able to follow this guide mentioned below, you should be able to transition from your regular to a vegan diet very easily:

Educate yourself

Starting a vegan diet is something that most people look into when they are looking to get healthy and feel their best. When you are learning about wellness about a plant-based diet, it is important that you go online and learn about it. You will find a lot of information on the internet, thanks to the growing popularity for this type of diet.

While people try this lifestyle as a trend, there are more that adopt this lifestyle for sustainability, animal, and health purposes. There are a lot of ways to educate yourself on the benefits of a vegan diet and smarter ways of doing so.

It is very important that you rely on the facts. In contrast to popular beliefs, most health sites and blogs do not largely state facts about the nutrition level – they are mostly another person's take on nutrition or someone else's trend or beliefs.

If you are looking for facts, it is suggested that you turn to organizations, holistic health practitioners, certified nutritionists, and registered dieticians. Via these sources, you will learn the exact nutrients from a vegan diet. You will also understand which foods will provide you with the most nutrition in easy-to-assimilate amounts.

Lastly, read more from more than a single reliable source, especially when it comes to nutrition. This is because you will find many different variations of single research. While the end result might be the same, each type of diet may work differently from one person to another.

Replace meat with delicious and Filling plant-based foods

Now, the good news is that you are trying to eat a vegan/vegetarian dish; on the other hand, the bad news is that you will miss all your favorite meat products. Nevertheless, going vegan does not mean that you will have to sacrifice the dishes that you loved eating. Almost everything you used to eat can be made with plant-based ingredients, even the meatiest dishes like Buffalo wings, meatballs, and burgers. All you need to do is make use of your creativity and imagination.

For instance, you can make use of TVP, Seitan, tempeh, and tofu to replace your meat products. While they may have the same texture as meat, they are actually plantbased and made from soybeans – Seitan is made from wheat-gluten, TVP (texturized vegetable protein) is made from vegetable protein, etc. With the help of these plantbased options, you can easily replace the meat in your regular meat dishes.

Tofu is considered the perfect replacement for chicken; for instance, you can use it in a chicken curry dish or traditional Chinese noodles. On the other hand, tempeh has a very flaky texture, which is wonderful for fish dishes like fish fillets and crab cakes; they can also be used to replace ground beef for tacos and meatballs.

Lastly, there is a wide range of alternatives that you can use to replace meat like jackfruit, eggplant, lentils, beans, and legumes. Apart from being great meat substitutes, they are also filled with a lot of nutrients so that you do not miss out on anything.

Learn new recipes

One of the best ways to switch to a plant-based diet is to ditch the meat and learn new recipes. It is important that you start immediately. You need to focus on enjoying seasonal produce like bright salads, instead of simply waiting for your dinner. Apart from the recipes mentioned above, you can also some others that you can find on the internet.

For instance, a bowl of zucchini-mushroom Caprese is a great choice. This dish is your farmer's market bounty that has come alive. It contains all the classic vegetables like basil, spinach, mushrooms, and fresh zucchini, all mixed to create this Italian masterpiece. Additionally, it does not contain more than 300 calories.

For more simplicity, you can opt for a simple apple quinoa power bowl. This is an autumn-inspired bowl that combines plant proteins from tofu and quinoa and also adds leafy greens and apples for that perfect balance of macro-nutrients you are looking for. This dish will keep you satisfied and full. Additionally, it is also quite easy to make – all you need to do is cook the quinoa and top it with your choice of greens like romaine, kale, and spinach. In the end, you need to add chopped apples and tofu cubes. For more taste varieties, you can add a tangy dressing.

If you want to start your day right, you can do so with a bowl of savory turmeric oats with tempeh bacon. This oat bowl will mix in all the flavors of turmeric, along with the goodness of tempeh bacon. Turmeric is known to have antioxidant and anti-inflammatory properties while oat will provide your body with a soluble fiber known as beta-glucan. This dish is full of minerals and vitamins from the greens (kale, Swiss chard, baby spinach, etc.).

Similar to these three recipes, you will find a lot of plantbased recipes online. All you need to do is look for it or make use of the recipes we have mentioned in the previous sections.

Shop for the right products

When you are new to the plant-based diet routine, you need to understand what types of products and ingredients you need to choose. You need to adopt a sustainable eating habit that will reduce land used and water consumption used for factory farming, reduce greenhouse gas emissions, etc., all of which contribute to environmental degradation and global warming.

Additionally, reducing the number of animal products in your diet and purchasing local produces will help drive the economy and reduces dependency on factory farming.

Right from breakfast products like bacon and eggs to dinner produces like steaks – most people tend to focus on them for meals. When you switch from this to a plantbased diet, your meals need to revolve around plant-based ingredients.

Some whole-foods that you need to look for include:

- **Beverages**: Sparkling water, tea, coffee, etc.

- **Plant-based protein**: Tempeh, tofu, and other plant-based powders and sources with no artificial ingredients or added sugar

- **Condiments**: Lemon juice, vinegar, soy sauce, nutritional yeast, mustard, salsa, etc.

- **Seasonings, herbs, and spices**: Salt, black pepper, turmeric, rosemary, basil, etc.

- **Unsweetened plant-based milk**: Cashew milk, almond milk, coconut milk, etc.

- **Nut butter, nuts, and seeds**: Tahini, natural peanut butter, sunflower seeds, pumpkin seeds, macadamia nuts, cashews, almonds, etc.

- **Legumes**: Black beans, peanuts, lentils, chickpeas, peas, etc.

- **Healthy fats**: Unsweetened coconut, coconut oil, olive oil, avocados, etc.

- **Whole grains**: Barley, brown rice pasta, quinoa, farro, rolled oats, brown rice, etc.

- **Starchy vegetables**: Butternut squash, sweet potatoes, potatoes, etc.

- **Vegetables**: Peppers, asparagus, carrots, cauliflower, broccoli, tomatoes, spinach, kale, etc.

- **Fruits**: Bananas, pineapple, peaches, pears, citrus fruits, berries, etc.

Cook simple dishes

Cooking vegetarian food is very easy; additionally, cooking these meatless meals will really satisfy your taste buds. Even if you have a party with non-vegetarians, you can easily serve simple vegetarian dishes. There are a lot of secrets to why cooking simple vegetarian dishes are so important.

Simple cooking also means that food needs to be balanced. You have to remember that combining fiber and protein in your meals will help you feel full for longer. As mentioned in the turmeric rice recipe above, you can easily get fiber and proteins from this dish.

Slow roasting is another simple way to cook vegetarian dishes. When you slow cook your food, you remove all the unwanted water, which makes the texture more chewable and also intensifies the overall flavor.

Your dish should also contain chewy ingredients. There are many chewy foods that you can eat and feed others like nuts, grilled mushrooms, and seared firm tofu. While cooking these foods may take some time and effort, they will make you feel full and offer the daily dose of ingredients you require.

For simple dishes, always remember to add some umami ingredients. This term was coined by the Japanese and roughly translates to delicious. These ingredients will enhance the overall flavor of the food. While it is new, it is definitely safe and occurs only naturally. Some vegetables that are high in umami content include onions, corn, peas, seaweed, tomatoes, and asparagus.

Eat whole foods and vegetables

When you are planning to adopt a plant-based diet, it is obvious that you will have to include whole vegetables and fruits in your diet. They contain vitamins, minerals, and good for your health, and protect you from a wide range of diseases.

If you are looking for a regular well-balanced diet for an active and healthy lifestyle, you should eat more vegetables and fruits. There are many types of fruits and vegetables that you can prepare in different styles. It is recommended that you eat at least five servings of vegetables and two portions of fruits each day.

Vegetables and fruits contain a lot of minerals and vitamins that are good for your health. Some of the nutrients include folic acid, phosphorus, zinc, magnesium, and Vitamins A, C, and E. Folic acid helps reduce blood levels of homocysteine, a substance that may prove to be a risk factor for coronary heart diseases.

Vegetables and fruits are low in sugar, salt, and fat. They are also considered a good source of dietary fiber. Apart from helping you maintain an active lifestyle, a well balanced and healthy intake of vegetables and fruits will help you reduce and maintain a healthy weight and lower your blood pressure and cholesterol levels.

Whole vegetables and fruits contain plant chemicals, or phytochemicals, which are biologically-active substances that protect you from different types of diseases. According to research, if you consume vegetables and fruits daily, you will lower the risk of high blood pressure (hypertension), cancer (some forms), heart diseases, stroke, and Type-2 diabetes.

Opt for good fats

Fat is a type of nutrients like carbohydrate and protein. It is important for your body to protect the health of your brain and heart and also absorb vitamins. Most of us have grown with the misconception that fats will raise your cholesterol level, add inches to your waistline, and cause a wide range of health problems. However, this fact is not accurate.

There are two types of fats – good fats and bad fats. Bad fats include saturated fats and artificial trans fats, which can cause a wide range of problems like an increased risk to certain diseases, clogged arteries, weight gain, etc. On the other hand, good fats consist of omega-3 fatty acids and unsaturated rats, which have opposite effects.

Healthy fats will help you control your weight, stay on top of your mental and physical health, and also manage your moods.

There are several benefits of good fats like:

- Preventing the narrowing and hardening of the arteries (atherosclerosis)

- Lowering blood pressure

- Lowering triglycerides, which is often associated with fighting inflammation and various heart diseases

- Preventing abnormal rhythms of the heart

- Increasing good HDL cholesterol and lowering bad LDL levels

- Lowering the risk of a stroke and heart disease

  Some great sources of monosaturated fat include:

- Peanut butter

- Nuts (cashews, pecans, macadamia, peanuts, almonds)

- Olives

- Avocados

- Oils like sesame, peanut, canola, and olive oil

Some good sources of polyunsaturated fat include:

- Tofu

- Soymilk

- Safflower and soybean oil

- Walnuts

- Flaxseed

- Pumpkin, sesame, and sunflower seeds

Eat fruit for dessert

Eating fruits for dessert is perhaps the best way to finish your meal without jeopardizing your diet. As mentioned above, fruits contain a lot of different nutrients that are beneficial for your health. Instead of eating pastries and ice cream, which are made from dairy products, you can easily create a delicious plate of fruity desserts that will cut down calories and replenish your body.

For instance, strawberries are fruits that every person loves – whether they are vegetarians, vegans, or meat eaters. They are considered the best options for health maintenance and weight loss. They are also sweet, refreshing, and filled with antioxidants like Vitamin C and lycopene, and fiber.

Another popular choice is bananas, which are high in nutrients like manganese, potassium, Vitamin B6, and fiber. When you are hungry, you can immediately eat a banana to replenish your body and refresh your vitality. Bananas have also proven to be an effective blood pressure reducer and appetite suppressor. It is recommended that you eat at least one, two hours before your main meal.

Bananas are considered some of the creamiest ingredients that can be used instead of heavily milk-based concoctions as a low-calorie alternative. A single medium-sized banana consists of about 100 calories, with a fiber value of 4-gms. A fully-ripened banana can be used as a substitute for buttercream. They also pair extremely well with other ingredients like honey, raisins, blueberries, and walnuts.

Similar to the above, there are several other delicious fruits that you can consume alone or pair up for a scrumptious dessert. They will prove to be beneficial for your health and help you avoid dairy products as well, something that is commonly seen in desserts today.

CHAPTER 4

PLANT-BASED NUTRITION TIPS FOR THE KIDS

It is not a surprise to see so many parents around the world that are raising children on plant-based diets. Most people that are new to this are concerned whether kids can be fed food that is completely plant-based and whether the foods are adequate for their normal growth. However, it has been studied that a well-planned vegetarian or vegan diet is perfect for people from all age groups.

Yes, it only makes sense that a certain health-promoting diet that is good for adults is also beneficial for children. Of course, the key here is planning. If you want to make sure that your kids are getting their daily dose of nutrients they require a wide range of ingredients like seeds, nuts, legumes, whole grains, vegetables, and fruits. As for nutrients that are difficult to obtain from plant foods like Vitamin B12 and D, you can make use of supplements and can be added to almond milk, soy, and other breakfast cereals.

Whether you want your child to eat plant-based food or eat any animal-based meals, this is a decision that is best left to you and your family members. Ensure that you explain your decision to your child's teachers, caretakers, friends, and relatives so that they understand the reason why you have made this choice.

How do you plant for different stages?

A child goes through different life stages before maturing into adulthood. You will have to plan your child's diet according to these stages mentioned below:

Infants

Once your infant stops weaning, they can be introduced to iron-fortified cereals like rice and then later move to different oat and barley varieties. You can prepare these dishes with soy formula or breast milk. Add pure vegetable and fruit purees like bananas, pears, peaches, applesauce, peas, carrots, and sweet potatoes.

After your child crosses the eight-month mark, you can start introducing crackers and dry bread, as well as proteins; quinoa, lentils or mashed beans, and mashed tofu are viable plant-based options.

Children between the ages of 1 and 4

During the early phases of childhood, children start enjoying certain plant-based products like mashed potatoes, bread, carrot sticks, fruits, rice, pasta, and oatmeal. During this age, it is recommended that you introduce your kids to a few flavors and tastes – however, ensure that you do not overwhelm or over-complicate them during their meals. Some great meal ideas for this age group include:

- *Breakfast:*

- Healthy pancakes with sliced fruits

- Oatmeal sweetened with raisins and applesauce

- Whole-grain cereal with rice milk and soy

- Fresh fruit salad

- *Lunch:*

- Beans and vegetable soup

- Corn tortillas filled with salsa and mashed beans

- Whole wheat pitas with bean dip or hummus

- Wholegrain bread sandwiches with tahini, sliced avocado, and hummus

- *Dinner:*

- Plant proteins like vegetable burgers, tofu, lentils, and well-cooked beans

- Whole grains and products like white grain bread, whole-wheat pasta, quinoa, and brown rice

- Sweet potato or mashed potato

- Steamed vegetables like broccoli, green beans, corn, peas, and carrots

- *Snacks:*

- Homemade baked goods

- Whole grain toast with jam or tahini

- Brown rice crackers

- Smoothies made of fruits

- Applesauce

- Celery and carrot sticks

- Freshly-sliced fruits

Children between the ages of 5 and 11

The foods mentioned in the above section are made primarily for that age group. By the time your kids reach this age group, you need to incorporate a greater variety of foods. A varied diet will ensure that your children meet all their nutritional needs; also, keep encouraging them to keep an open mind to try new dishes.

You can introduce new types of plant-based foods to your kid's repertoire like different types of vegetables, legumes, and grains. You can also include different types of cuisines like the Mediterranean, Mexican, and Asia. While your kids may not like it at first, they will eventually get used to the texture and taste of the new food.

Additionally, you can also get your kids involved with the cooking process, as they will be able to help around by shopping for the ingredients or look for the recipes. This way, they will learn all about the flavors of the food and eat healthily in an engaging and fun way.

You need to recreate familiar foods that your kids love and create their plant-based versions like joes made of lentils instead of ground meat, cheese-less pizza, vegetable burgers, etc. You can also keep the lunchboxes interesting and fresh by adding different types of sandwich fillings, healthy homemade baked items, and vegetable/fruit snacks.

When it comes to birthdays, you do not have to overthink! You can offer them baked tortilla chips with salsa, raw vegetables with delicious plant-based sides, fresh fruit skewers, and even burgers and hot dogs that are made of vegetable meat substitutes. Additionally, there are also many birthday recipes that you can create with plantbased ingredients that can also be used to create dishes that your children can take to their school events and share with their friends.

Children above the age of 12

By this age, your children will probably start eating the same foods that you are; however, they may need to eat at more intervals than you. If your kid is raised in a vegan home environment, the transition to proper plant-based home meals will be smooth. All you need to do is remove highly processed items from your home and replace them with healthier options.

However, if you plan on switching to a 'standard' home diet, it is wise to discuss it with your kids. While your children may be interested in environmental issues, animal ethics, and overall healthy eating, there are more chances of them thinking that you are trying to ruin their lives. If the latter scenario takes place, it is advised that you make some compromises and have them try out vegan versions of animal-based foods like vegan cheeses, burgers, lunch meats, and vegetable 'chicken' chunks.

As your children are growing up, it would prove to be mutually beneficial for you to get them involved in the decision making when it comes to meals. Ask them what they would like to eat for lunch or have them decide the menu for dinner. If they are prepared and interested in cooking, you can allow them to prepare plant-based recipes for the family once in a blue moon.

CHAPTER 5

PLANT-BASED NUTRITION TIPS FOR THE ELDERLY

We are all growing older; this means that you will have to keep a close eye on some bodily changes that will eventually occur. First, your sensitivity will start decreasing and your senses may not feel as strong as it once did. Among these is the loss of taste and smell, which will decrease your appetite. Other changes include macular degeneration, physical difficulties, memory loss, etc.

Via all these changes, it could eventually lead to depression. Thankfully, keeping a close eye on the foods you eat and switching to a plant-based diet will help you prevent all these problems. However, switching from your previous diet, including a vegetarian diet, to a plantbased diet sans the need for dairy products is not going to be easy.

The first aspect of the matter is to maintain your protein intake. Senior adults require more proteins than other age groups to maintain normal body function, preserve lean body mass, and upkeep their overall health. While most young and middle-aged adults need only 0.75g of protein per kilogram per day, healthy senior adults require a daily protein intake of 1-1.2g per kilogram of body weight. For older adults with severe illness or are malnourished, this amount is even higher; if not, it could result in a hyper metabolic state, where your body would require more protein and energy to function.

To ensure that you get an adequate amount of proteins, you need to ensure that your snacks and meals contain plant-based proteins like nut butter, seeds and nuts, wild rice, quinoa, lentils, kidney beans, black-eyed beans, tofu, and chickpeas. As for yogurt and milk, you can make use of soya alternatives.

The meals also need to contain Vitamin D and calcium, both of which play important roles in maintaining the health of the old bones. Senior adults often complain about fractures and osteoporosis, which are major causes of mortality in them.

While young adults require 700mg of calcium per day, men and women over the age of 55 (or past menopause, for women) require 1200mg of calcium each day. There is a wide range of non-dairy products that contain calcium like white bread, pita bread, calcium-fortified cereals, and fortified almond and soy milk.

As for Vitamin D, senior adults require about 10mcg of this nutrient every day. Apart from supporting bone health, it also supports the proper functioning of the immune system. This is quite important for older adults because they are more vulnerable to Vitamin D deficiency as they may not be as exposed to sunlight or their skin is no longer able to synthesize Vitamin D.

Some great sources of Vitamin D include dairy alternatives, breakfast cereals, fortified spreads, and sunlight.

However, acquiring Vitamin D from the diet is simply not enough, especially during winters. Hence, it is recommended that you take a supplement of 10mcg per day; for vegans, you can opt for lichen-derived Vitamin D3 and Vitamin D2 as they are not derived from animal sources.

For older adults, getting their daily dose of Vitamin B12 is also very important. This vitamin is needed for the production of red blood cells, providing energy, and keeping the nervous system healthy. Both young and old adults require 1.5mcg of Vitamin B12 each day. However, procuring this vitamin is not easy for people that follow a strictly plant-based diet.

This is because the vitamin is mostly found in animal based products like eggs, fish, and meat. However, some plant-based alternatives for Vitamin B12 include nondairy milk, soya yogurt, yeast extracts (like Marmite), and fortified breakfast cereals. While taking less than 2mg of B12 each day will mostly not cause any harm, you must get it checked with a registered dietician first.

The lack of iron can pose to be a potential problem for men and women above the age of 65 years. Iron is an important requirement by the body and is needed to produce red blood cells to carry oxygen from one part of the body to another. It also enhances physical performance, development, and functioning of cognitive and thyroid metabolism supports the immune system and promotes faster wound healing. On average, senior adults require about 8.7mg of iron each day.

There are several plant sources that are rich in iron like dried fruits, pulses, seeds, spinach, and other leafy vegetables and whole grains. Since iron from plant sources is not absorbed as effectively as iron from animal-based foods, you can also include products like broccoli, green pepper, and citrus fruits that are rich in Vitamin C so that iron can be absorbed much easier.

Lastly, ensure that every bite that you take counts. For older people, it is natural to find the appetite decrease as they get older. There are several reasons that contribute to this fact – difficulties in swallowing and/or chewing, impaired senses of smell, vision and taste, acute illnesses, and constipation.

This reduced diet contributes to nutritional deficiencies and unintentional weight loss. Hence, it is always important that all the required nutrition is present in the food that you eat, especially if it is a plant-based diet.

If you can manage to follow through with the abovementioned ways to increase the absorption of nutrients via a plant-based diet, you will gain a lot of benefits. Some of them include:

Slow down the aging process

According to studies, it has been confirmed that plantbased foods are more effective at reversing the aging process, as compared to animal-based diets. Plant-based diets include foods that increase the levels of telomerase, which is the enzyme that helps rebuild the telomeres of the human DNA after it dies. Once the telomeres expire, we die.

Looking younger

It has been reported that older people improve their skin conditions and complexions when they switch to a plant-based diet. This is because these foods contain antioxidants that eliminate free radicals from the skin, thereby preventing premature aging. In short, you will look and may even feel younger, as this diet will heal skin tissues and moisturize your skin.

Increase energy levels

When you switch to a plant-based diet, you will be provided with more energy that will help you complete more tasks during the day or increase your exercising levels. Since plant-based foods are easier to break down, as compared to animal-based products like dairy and meat, you will have more energy to spend throughout the day.

CHAPTER 6

TIPS TO INCREASE NUTRITION ABSORPTION FROM YOUR PLANT-BASED DIET

Throughout our lives, we have repeatedly been reminded to eat as many greens as possible. 'Eat your carrots; it will improve your eyesight' – does it sound familiar? Plantbased foods like vegetables and fruits are packed with different types of nutrients like minerals and vitamins that are required by the body to function optimally. However, what most people are unable to understand is the difference between eating healthy foods and your body's ability to absorb the nutrients.

It is possible that you eat a healthy and nutritious plantbased diet; however, you may not feel more energized or healthy, which can only feel discouraging. The thing here is that your body is not absorbing the nutrient, even if you are eating the correct foods.

Why is your body not absorbing the nutrients?

There are a lot of different factors that influence your body's ability to absorb nutrients; some important ones include genetics, psychological stress, lifestyle habits, diet, age, and also your gut microbiome. These factors play important roles when it comes to the absorption of minerals and vitamins by your body.

What is nutrient absorption?

As most of us already know, the food that we eat goes into our stomachs; however, this is just a small part of the overall digestive process. Once inside your gut, the gut microbiome and digestive enzymes will start working to break the food down into smaller particles for easy absorption.

From the stomach, the food molecules then travel to the upper portion of the small intestines and then move throughout the body via the bloodstream. This is an important process since the absorption of nutrients will vary significantly.

It has been studied that the body can absorb as little as 10% or optimally 90%. It is important that you understand your body's capability to absorb nutrients because how your body will carry out the daily tasks will depend on this fact.

If your body is unable to absorb the nutrients, it could lead to a lot of different physical and mental problems.

Reading the labels

You should know that the nutritional levels you see on the packaging of the food will never give you a complete picture. While you must read the labels, you will never understand the entire spectrum of the nutrients that the product contains; there are several reasons for this – the way the dates are arranged, the natural variability of the product, the serving size, etc.

For example, you may read that a single banana contains approximately 398mg of potassium. However, the banana you eat during your lunch break may feel inadequate. This is because the information that you have read is an estimate based on the different types of bananas within the range of 360 and 502mg.

Adding modern lifestyle into the mix, these figures become very vague. Unless you have something that will analyze how much nutrients are getting absorbed by your body, it is almost impossible to figure the absorption quantity each time you eat.

Tips to increase nutrition absorption by your body

The overall digestion and absorption process is a very complex one. There are a lot of different functions involved, with different organs working simultaneously to produce saliva, enzymes, bile, acid, etc. Here are some tips that will help you increase the nutrition absorbing capabilities of your body:

Slow eating

The first trick in the book is to stop eating fast. As most of us already know, the digestion process starts with chewing; this act releases several types of enzymes that start breaking the food for the complex digestion process later. It has been studied by medical experts that chewing your food at least 40 times will help you absorb more nutrients than chewing only ten times. Slow eating and proper chewing will make nutrients to become more accessible.

Reduce your stress

Most people tend to experience unpleasant bowel symptoms when they get stressed out. This happens because the body redirects the energy that is required for digestion to help you deal with stress and anxiety. Hence, you must prioritize self-care. It is recommended that you do not think about anything stressful just before you start to eat. Always allow yourself time and space to cook your food; additionally, ensure that you sit and eat your food.

Boost your gut health

As mentioned above, your gut health will dictate how well your body can absorb the nutrients. The gut is known as the primary nutrient absorption center of the body; hence, it is important that you take care of the bacteria and ensure that they are healthy. According to studies, it has been found that more than 30% of the carbs and proteins enter the colon undigested; this is where the bacteria come in to break them down.

You can increase the health of your gut by eating food that the bacteria love, like vegetables with high dietary fiber and fermented foods. Also, you can try a probiotic supplement like vegan and non-GMO capsules.

Hydrate

One of the most important factors that can make or break out digestion is hydration. When your body does not get enough water or fluids, the results can be seen in the stools. The human digestive system is dependent on the level of hydration as it is not possible for the blood to transport nutrients throughout the body, without enough water.

Foods that promote nutrition absorption

Of course, changing your lifestyle is important; however, the core idea behind nutrition absorption will start with the foods that you eat. You must focus on the right food pairings. While some raw fruits and vegetables may not provide as much nutrition as you may look for, pairing them with different foods will allow them to work cohesively to improve your body's absorption capabilities.

Vitamin C and Iron

It is not easy for the human body to absorb iron from food. Hence, you need to pair iron-rich foods, like spinach, with anything rich in Vitamin C, like sweet yellow peppers, chili peppers, acerola cherries, or herbs like thyme and parsley.

It has been studied that Vitamin C strengthens your body's capability to absorb nutrients (iron, in this case). There are several recipes that pair iron-rich plant foods with plant-based foods that are rich in Vitamin C.

Fatty acids and fat-soluble vitamins

The term 'fat-soluble' refers to vitamins like E, K, D, and A that need fatty acids to be absorbed by the body. Hence, when you are eating a plant-based diet (most plants contain these vitamins), you need to pair them with healthy plant-based fats, which can be found in produces like avocados, seeds, and nuts.

Opt for a smoothie

Yes, a fruit smoothie or daily juice will increase sugar consumption; however, consuming fruits in this form will help your body absorb nutrients more effectively. As per studies, it has been found that fiber found in whole fruits may bind to certain micronutrients, which makes it difficult for the small intestines to absorb. Hence, consuming in the juice/smoothie form will allow it to get absorbed more easily. However, it is important to understand that moderation is the key; always look for food recipes that are delicious, easy to make, and fun.

Tomatoes and olive oil

Tomatoes contain lycopene, which is an effective antioxidant that fights off various diseases. Additionally, lycopene is also known to prevent certain types of cancers, like prostate cancer. When you cook tomatoes, you can add some olive oil, which helps the body increase its lycopene absorption capabilities. You can also drizzle the oil on baked tomatoes or whip up a tomato sauce with olive oil. Or, you can combine different ingredients for a simple summer grain bowl.

Turmeric and black pepper

If you love spicy stir-fries, then it is common to use turmeric as a flavoring agent. In fact, it has been used for centuries; apart from the delicious flavor, turmeric is also known for its powerful anti-inflammatory properties that make it a powerful antioxidant. According to experts, the spice is beneficial for kidney health and also relieves some symptoms of arthritis. When you use black pepper along with turmeric, the beneficial compounds become more bio-available and will provide you with maximum benefits. Additionally, the taste improves a lot as well!

Chickpeas or beans with rice

Individually, each one of these components provides various health benefits. However, you can expect some unknown perks if you combine all these foods together. Chickpeas and beans are packed with fiber and proteins, which makes them perfect to accompany starchy foods like rice. With the help of chickpeas/beans, your body will be able to regulate the levels of carbohydrates and prevent unwanted spikes in the blood sugar level. The overall meal will be well-balanced.

Apart from the above, there are many other similar combinations that will increase the nutrition absorption capabilities of your body for maximum health benefits. However, it is just as important that you read about these combos, instead of simply trying them directly.

CHAPTER 7

12 PLANT-BASED RECIPES

Now that we have gone through the scientific aspects of plant-based diets, let us get into the section that we absolutely love! Yes, we are talking about the recipe section.

Below, we have listed down some simple plant-based recipes that you can use to whip up any type of meal within some time. All these ingredients can be found easily near your local store and the cooking aspect is not so difficult as well.

Breakfast

If you are looking for some delicious plant-based breakfast, you can easily learn these recipes mentioned below:

Orange French toast

This particular French toast recipe makes use of aquafaba, cinnamon, and orange zest to create thick and soft toast. The highlight of the job is aquafaba, which makes the dish very egg-ish. Aquafaba is a liquid that comes out after cooking or soaking legumes or cooking beans.

The liquid is very thick and often used as an egg substitute. The proteins and starches make it perfect for foaming, emulsifying, binding, or thickening dishes. While you have the choice of purchasing aquafaba, you can also create your own.

Ingredients:

For the French toast:

- Whole grain bread slices (3/4-inches thickness, 8)

- Orange zest (1/2 tablespoon)

- Salt (2 pinches, optional)

- Ground cinnamon (1/4 teaspoon)

- Pure maple syrup (2 tablespoons)

- Aquafaba (1 cup)

- Almond flour (1/2 cup)

- Plant milk (Unflavored and unsweetened, 1-1/2 cup)

For the Berry compote:

- Pure maple syrup (1 teaspoon)

- Applesauce (1/2 cup)

- Raspberries or blueberries (thawed, frozen, or fresh, 4.5-ounces)

Instructions:

You need to begin by preheating the oven up to 200°C; once done, you can put a wire rack on top of the baking sheet. After this, you can combine the rest of the ingredients like salt, cinnamon, maple syrup, aquafaba, flour, and plant milk in another bowl and keep mixing it until the result becomes smooth and consistent. Move the mixture to a shallow pan, add the orange zest, and mix well.

 Next, start warming a non-stick skillet over medium heat and dip the bread into the mixture that you have prepared. Let the sticks sit for some seconds and keep turning them. Place the breadsticks into the skillet and cook the bread for some minutes on both sides until it is brown.

Place the toasted bread on the wire rack and bake it in the oven for 10-15 minutes; this will make them crispy. While the bread is being baked, you can start adding the maple syrup, applesauce, and berries into the mixture and let it run until it reaches a chunky consistency. Serve the bread with the berry compote.

Banana almond granola

Granola is one of those dishes that can prove to be a delicious snack and you can gouge on them without feeling guilty. This dish is quite a simple and delicious breakfast; in fact, you will be very surprised to learn that this oilfree dish can turn out to be so crunchy. You can cook the dish in advance and store it for future consumption too. You will be able to avoid store-bought granola that often contains preservatives, additives, unhealthy fats, and high sugar content.

Ingredients:

- Almonds (Slivered, toasted, 1 cup)
- Salt (1 teaspoon)
- Almond extract (1 teaspoon)
- Bananas (Peeled and chopped, 2)
- Dates (Pitted and chopped, 2 cups)
- Rolled oats (8 cups)

Instructions:

You need to begin by preheating the oven to 135°C. Then, add the oats to a large bowl and line two 13x18inch baking sheets with parchment paper. Lay down the dates on a medium-sized saucepan and add a cup of water for boiling. Let the dates cook for 10 minutes and keep adding water so that the dates do not stick to the pan.

Remove the dates and add them into a blender, along with salt, almond extract, and bananas; blend them until the mixture becomes creamy and smooth.

Add the mixture to the oats and mix them well. Divide the granola between the baking sheets and spread them out evenly. Bake them in the oven for about an hour, switching sides every 10 minutes. Once the granola becomes crispy, you can remove them and let it cool. Once done, you can add the slivered almonds. You can store the granola in an airtight container.

Chickpea Omelet

If you want to have a great day ahead, an omelet is considered the best breakfast dish. However, if you are a vegan, then this option is off the table. However, it is possible to create an egg-free omelet with simple ingredients and flavorings like nutritional yeasts, chickpea flour, etc.

The chickpea omelet is the best option for a vegan breakfast because it is egg-free, soy-free, gluten-free, and vegan. However, the taste and texture of the dish are surprisingly similar to an egg omelet. If you have not cooked with chickpea flour, you will love to try out this recipe. The cooking is very easy.

Additionally, you can also add some plant-delicious toppings like hot sauce, spinach, tomatoes, etc. Another great aspect of this chickpea omelet is that it can be served as breakfast, lunch, or dinner. Cooking this dish should not take more than 30 minutes and can be chowed down within seconds.

Ingredients:

- Sautéed mushrooms (4 ounces, optional)

- Green onions (Chopped, green and white parts, 3)

- Baking soda (1/2 teaspoon)

- Nutritional yeast (1/3 cup)

- Black pepper (1/4 teaspoon)

- White pepper (1/4 teaspoon)

- Garlic powder (1/2 teaspoon)

- Onion powder (1/2 teaspoon)

- Chickpea flour (1 cup)

Instructions:

In a small bowl, you need to add baking soda, nutritional yeast, black pepper, white pepper, garlic powder, onion powder, and chickpea flour. Add a cup of water and keep mixing it until the batter becomes smooth.

Heat a frying pan and pour the batter into it, similar to how you would make pancakes. Sprinkle the mushrooms and green onions into the mix as the 'omelet' cooks. Keep flipping the omelet to cook on both sides.

Once done, you can serve this chickpea omelet with whatever you like – hot sauce, salsa, spinach, and/or tomatoes.

Polenta with pears and cranberries

This particular polenta recipe is another easy breakfast recipe that you can eat in the morning. It is quite a crowd favorite and will quickly become your favorite too! To create this stunning breakfast, you do not require a lot of things – just the ripest pears you can find in the market like D'anjou, Asian, and Bosc. Additionally, you can choose fresh cranberries according to the ongoing season.

Another fun aspect of this polenta with pears and cranberries recipe is that it can also be served as a scrumptious dessert. The cooked fruit on top of the butter-like polenta is the best combination.

Ingredients:

- Basic polenta (basic, kept warm)

- Ground cinnamon (1 teaspoon)

- Cranberries (Dried or fresh (1 cup)

- Pears (Diced, cored, or peeled, 2)

- Brown rice syrup (1/4 cup)

Instructions:

Heat the brown rice syrup in a saucepan. Once sufficiently heated up, you can add cinnamon, cranberries, and pears into the mix. Keep mixing and stirring until the pears become tender.

Once done, you can serve the polenta in different bowls and add this pear compote for added flavors.

Lunch

Lunch is a very important meal of the day. Hence, you need to ensure that you eat some quality food so that you have

Spicy Buffalo Chickpea Wraps

If you love spicy food, then these buffalo chickpea wraps are the best choice for you. The overall recipe is very easy and will give your taste buds a thrilling experience. These wraps are spicy, savory, and hearty. The crunchy element of the dish comes from the vegetables and the tenderness from the chickpeas.

If you are looking for a satisfying but quick lunch, this dish is considered the perfect option. Apart from being delicious, it also contains healthy fibers and proteins. Additionally, you can also create your blend of dressings and toppings.

Ingredients:

- Sea salt (1 pinch)

- Garlic powder (4 tablespoons)

- Hot sauce (4 tablespoons)

- Coconut oil or olive oil (1 tablespoon)

- Chickpeas (Rinsed, drained, and dried, 1 15-ounce can)

- Romaine lettuce (Roughly chopped)

- Hot water (1-2 tablespoons)

- Lemon

- Maple syrup (1-1/2 tablespoon)

- Hummus (1/3 cup)

- Vegan-friendly flatbread, pita, or flour (3-4)

Instructions:

To create the dressings, you need to add lemon juice, maple syrup, and hummus into a whisking bowl and keep mixing until it becomes thick; you can also add hot water for thickness. Keep adjusting the flavor according to your taste and then add the romaine lettuce.

As for the chickpeas, you need to drain and dry them into a separate bowl. Add the hot sauce and coconut/olive oil, salt, and garlic powder and toss them together. Heat a skillet and add the chickpeas for some minutes; later, mash them with a spoon.

Once the chickpeas are dried out and hot, you can add the remaining sauce. Stir and mix them properly. As for the assembly, you can top each wrap with the romaine salad and chickpeas. For added flavors, you can also add onion, avocado, and/or tomatoes.

Collard Green Spring Rolls, with Sunflower Butter Dipping Sauce

These spring rolls are colorful and healthy dishes that you can make within 30 minutes. They can be served for lunch and can also be eaten as side dishes. If you are into spring rolls, then there are a lot of varieties that you can choose like Thai spring rolls, quinoa spring rolls, Pad Thai spring rolls, etc. All of these can be prepared by the same method.

Ingredients:

For the sauce:

- Hot water
- Chili garlic sauce (1/2 teaspoon)
- Lime (Juiced, 2 tablespoons)
- Maple syrup (2-3 tablespoon)
- Tamari (1-1/2 tablespoon)
- Sunflower seed butter (Unsalted, 1/3 cup)

For the spring rolls:

- Carrots (3)
- Red or purple cabbage (Finely chopped, 1 cup)

- Packed basil (1 cup)

- Bean sprouts (1-1/2 cup)

- Red bell pepper (Sliced thinly, 1)

- Collard greens (1 bundle)

- Tofu (10 ounces)

Instructions:

With the help of a clean and absorbent towel, you need to clean the tofu and remove the excess liquid. As the tofu gets dried, you can start with the prep of the green collards; chop off the stems and trim down the thickness of the stems. While this step is not particularly needed, it will roll/fold more easily.

Prep the vegetables and then slice the tofu into rectangular cubes. Add the chili garlic sauce, lime juice, maple syrup, tamari, and sunflower seed butter to prepare the dipping sauce. Keep whisking them until you reach a thick consistency. Adjust the flavor according to your tastes.

Fill the collard with carrot, bean sprout, cabbage, red pepper, tofu, and basil. Fold the collard greens with your hands so that the fillings are secured and tuck in the sides.

Keep rolling the collard until you have a loose spring roll and lay it seam-side.

For serving, you can slice the rolls into half and service the dish with the dipping sauce. Or else, you can also leave them whole.

Roasted Rainbow Vegetable Bowl

This dish is a beautiful vegetable bowl that is very healthy and can be eaten for lunch. It can be prepared very easily and quickly, which makes it perfect for anyone who is always in a hurry. Additionally, roasting vegetables makes it easier for the digestion system and enhances the overall flavor of the dish. This vegetable bowl is colorful, satisfying, and wholesome, thereby making it a perfect dish for any type of meal.

Ingredients:

- Kale or collard greens (2 cups)

- Broccoli (1 cup)

- Red pepper (Thinly sliced, 1 cup)

- Cabbage (Thinly sliced, 1 cup)

- Sea salt (1/2 teaspoon)

- Curry powder (1 teaspoon)

- Melted coconut or avocado oil (2 tablespoons)

- Radishes (Medium-sized, 4)

- Beet (Medium-sized, 1)

- Carrots

- Sweet potato

- Yellow or red baby potatoes

Instructions:

Start by preheating the oven to 204°C and then line two baking sheets with parchment paper. On one of the baking sheets, you need to add sea salt, curry powder, and oil on radishes, beets, carrots, sweet potatoes, and potatoes. Keep tossing the mixture and let it bake for 2025 minutes.

Add broccoli, bell pepper, and cabbage on the second baking sheet and drizzle the reaming oil, sea salt, and curry powder. Toss the mixture properly.

Once the carrots and potatoes hit the 10-minute mark, add the second baking sheet and then bake the entire batch for 15-20 minutes. When you reach the last five minute mark, you can add the kale or collard greens to either roast or pan until bright green and tender. You can serve the dish with avocado and season it with sea salt, hemp seeds, tahini, or lemon juice.

Loaded Kale Salad

This is a hearty and healthy salad that can easily replace other types of unhealthy lunch options. It is filled with nutrients, thanks to the healthy ingredients. The dish is quite versatile and some ingredients can be swapped for other options like butternut squash, cornbread, etc. When it comes to a perfect lunch for a weekday, then beating this kale salad is quite hard.

Ingredients:

For the salad:

- Choice sprouts (1/2 cups)
- Hemp seeds (1/4 cups)
- Avocado (Cubed, 1)
- Cherry tomatoes (1/2 cup)
- Kale (8 cups)

For the dressing:

- Water (1/4 cup)
- Sea salt (1 pinch)
- Maple syrup (1-2 tablespoon)
- Lemon juice (2-3 tablespoon)
- Tahini (1/3 cup)

For the vegetables:

- Curry powder (Optional, ½ teaspoon)
- Sea salt (1 pinch)
- Water (2 tablespoons)
- Beet (Thinly sliced, 1)

- Carrots (Large, halved, 4)

- For the quinoa

- Water (360ml)

- Quinoa (Well-rinsed, 3/4 cups)

Instructions:

Rinse and strain the quinoa over a small pot and then toast it for a minute or two. Keep the quinoa under low heat until the liquid gets absorbed. Set the quinoa aside once cooked. Preheat the oven up to 190°C and add beets and carrots to the baking sheet. Add the oil/water and the seasonings and keep tossing the mixture. Roast the dish for another 30 minutes or until it becomes golden brown.

As the mixture is roasting in the oven, you can prepare the dressing by adding salt, maple syrup, lemon juice, and tahini. Add water and whisk until the consistency is smooth. Taste and adjust the flavor to your preferences.

Next, arrange the kale on the bowl or serving platter and top the dish with toppings like roasted vegetables, cooked quinoa, avocado, and tomatoes. Even if you are left with some leftovers, they can be eaten within the next three days.

Dinner

If you want to finish the day on a happy note, you need to ensure that your dinner is tasty. This meal needs to be light and easy to digest. Here are some recipes that you will absolutely love cooking and eating:

Sweet Potato Chickpea Buddha Bowl

This is a flavorful bowl that you can eat for dinner. The dish is sweet and savory, with subtle hints of spiciness. The food is extremely comforting and warm and will provide you with incredible satisfaction. Apart from being flavorful, it is also filled with a lot of health benefits. The dish is not heavy and will not cause you to sleep with a heavy stomach.

Ingredients:

For the chickpeas:

- Turmeric (Optional, 1/4 teaspoon)

- Oregano (Optional, 1/2 teaspoon)

- Salt and pepper (1/4 teaspoon)

- Garlic powder (3/4 teaspoon)

- Chili powder (3/4 teaspoon)

- Cumin (1 teaspoon)

- Chickpeas (5 ounces)

For the vegetables:

- Kale (Larger stems removed, 2)

- Broccoli (Chopped, 1 bundle)

- Sweet potatoes (Halved, 2)

- Red onion (Medium, 1/2)

- Avocado, olive, or melted coconut oil (2 tablespoons)

For the tahini sauce:

- Hot water (2-4 tablespoon)

- Lemon (Medium, 1/2)

- Maple syrup (1 tablespoon)

- Tahini (1/4 cup)

- Lemon (Juiced, 1/2 cup)

- Maple syrup (1 tablespoon)

- Hot water (2-4 tablespoon)

Instructions:

You can begin by preheating the oven to 204°C. On a bare baking sheet, you need to arrange the onions and sweet potatoes. Add some oil and ensure that the sweet potatoes are well-coated. The skin side needs to face the sheet. Bake them for ten minutes and then flip the sweet potatoes, while adding the broccolini. Drizzle some oil on the broccolini with salt and pepper.

After baking for another ten minutes, remove the dish from the oven and add the kale. Add oil, salt, and pepper to the kale and bake for five minutes and set it aside.

While the vegetables are being baked in the oven, you can heat a skillet and add chickpeas to a mixing bowl. You need to toss some seasonings on the chickpeas. Once the skillet becomes hot, you can add oil and the chickpeas and sauté and stir the mixture. Turn the heat down if the chickpeas are browning quickly. After the chickpeas are cooked, you need to set it aside.

As for the sauce, you can add the lemon juice, maple syrup, and tahini into a whisking bowl. Add some hot water and set it aside. For serving, slice the sweet potatoes into smaller sizes and top it up with the tahini sauce and chickpeas.

Cauliflower Rice Stir-Fry

This cauliflower rice stir-fry is a recipe that you can prepare and eat quickly. Additionally, it is also very satisfying, healthy, and perfect if you do not have a lot of money left to spend. The flavor is neutral and full of nutrients and fiber.

Ingredients:

For the sauce:

- Water (1-2 tablespoon)

- Maple syrup (1 tablespoon)

- Fresh ginger (Minced, 1/2 teaspoon)

- Chili garlic sauce

- Lime juice (2-4 teaspoon)

- Coconut aminos (4 tablespoons)

- Peanut butter or almond (2 tablespoons)

- Coconut oil or sesame oil (1 teaspoon)

For the cauliflower:

- Water (3 tablespoons)

- Cauliflower head

For the stir-fry:

- Toasted almonds or roasted cashews (1/2-3/4 cup)

- Green or red cabbage (1 cup)

- Green onions (1 cup)

- Pepper

- Coconut aminos (3 tablespoons)

- Green beans (1-1/2 tablespoon)

- Green beans (1-1/2 tablespoon)

- Coconut or sesame oil (1 tablespoon)

For the serving:

- Chili garlic sauce or sriracha

- Lime wedges

- Fresh cilantro

Instructions:

Wash the cauliflower and remove the greens. Then, cut the cauliflower into large chunks with a box grater. Remove excess water with a paper towel and sauté the rice and cauliflower mixture on a skillet. Cover the lid of the skillet and let the dish steam. Add seasoning as desired.

For the sauce, you need to add water, maple syrup, ginger, chili garlic sauce, lime juice, coconut aminos, peanut butter or almond, and oil into a mixing bowl; adjust the taste according to your preference. Heat a skillet and add the cauliflower rice and add the sauce into the mixture. Add green beans and keep tossing the mixture.

Keep cooking the mixture until it is well-combined. You can serve the dish with any other choice of sauce, lime wedges, or fresh cilantro. Additionally, the dish can also be kept up to three days in a refrigerator.

Vegan garlic pasta

You cannot go wrong with the vegan garlic pasta. This dish can be created within 30 minutes and is considered a perfect dinner dish; alternatively, you can also eat this dish for breakfast the next day. The ingredients are extremely simple and extremely healthy. The flavors are natural and you can add other types of seasonings to adjust the overall taste of the dish.

Ingredients:

- Lemon juice (1-2 tablespoon)
- Nutritional yeast (2-3 tablespoons)
- Almond breeze (Plain, unsweetened, 2-1/2 cups)
- All-purpose flour (Unbleached, 3-4 tablespoon)
- Sea salt and black pepper (1 pinch)
- Garlic (8 cloves)
- Shallots (Medium, 2)
- Olive oil
- Whole wheat pasta (10 ounces)
- Grape tomatoes (3 cups)

Instructions:

You can start by preheating the oven and preparing the baking sheet. Throw in the tomatoes with sea salt and olive oil. Bake the tomatoes for 20 minutes. In the meantime, you can start prepping the other ingredients.

Take a large pot, pour water into it, and start boiling the pasta. Set it aside once the pasta is done and drained. As for the sauce, you can heat a large skillet and start heating the oil. Add the pepper, salt, shallots, and garlic and keep stirring it until it smells nice and softens up.

Take the flour and start whisking it. Add the almond milk, nutritional yeast, salt, pepper, and bring it to simmer. For consistent thickness, keep cooking it for 4-5 minutes. For cheesier flavor, add nutritional yeast. As for the sauce, you can transfer it into a blender until the consistency is smooth and creamy. Add the seasonings according to your taste. Once done, it is ready to serve with the pasta.

Vegan 'pulled pork' sandwich

Ingredients:

- Water (2 tablespoons)
- Vegan barbeque sauce (3/4 cups)
- Garlic powder (1 teaspoon)
- Sea salt and pepper
- Paprika (Ground, 1-1/2 tablespoon)
- Organic brown sugar or coconut sugar
- Carrots (Grated or shredded, 1-1/2 cups)
- Yellow or white onion (Medium, 1/2)
- Green lentils (1 cup)
- Grapeseed or olive oil

Instructions:

Add the lentils and the water into a saucepan and heat it. Let it cook for 18 minutes, drain the excess water, and set it aside. On another skillet, add oil, seasonings, and onion and sauté for 4-5 minutes. Then add the water, barbeque sauce, garlic powder, paprika, coconut sugar, carrots, and lentils. Stir it for 5-10 minutes.

Keep adjusting the flavor according to your taste. Another optional choice is to blend half of the mixture and mix in some carrots and lentils; the texture will come out as more cohesive. Serve the mixture with some toasted buns, with toppings of your choice. On the sides, you can add sliced green onions, carrots, or shredded red cabbage.
For more flavor, you can add some extra barbeque sauce.

CONCLUSION

From the above, we now understand how important a plant-based and mucusless diet is for our overall health. While this type of diet has been at the center of different controversies, it does have a lot of followers. The overall idea of this diet is to consume foods that do not cause the production of mucus like leafy green vegetables, nuts, and fruits.

This theory was first conceptualized by Prof Arnold Ehret; he created the definition of what types of foods are included in this type of diet, along with flushing the digestive system with water. This type of diet will remove all toxins from your body and will control its natural balance. Some obvious benefits include weight loss and increased energy levels, without losing out on nutrition. As a matter of the fact, a mucusless diet goes beyond vegetarian and vegan diets, as mentioned at the start of the article.

When you first start with a mucusless/vegan diet, you will feel like your lungs have become much clearer than before. As soon as you start your diet, the toxins will be released back into your bloodstream. While you may feel sick and dizzy at first, you will feel a surge of energy passing through your veins.

Starting a mucusless diet is not difficult; all you need to do is start with fruits and vegetables, and the rest will follow automatically. The overall rule here is to eat anything that is vegetable- or fruit-based. If you are able to stick with this type of diet, you should start to see the results in the following weeks.

With the help of this article, you will feel more encouraged to try out this type of diet; in fact, there is nothing wrong with trying out this type of diet. You can make use of the recipes mentioned above to try out new dishes that will not make you miss out on your animal-based foods. Give this diet a go!

CPSIA information can be obtained
at www.ICGtesting.com
Printed in the USA
BVHW011801270522
638300BV00007B/166